STRANGE
BODIES

Also by Tom de Freston
from Granta Books

Wreck: A Story of Art and Survival

STRANGE BODIES

A Story of Loss and Desire

TOM DE FRESTON

GRANTA

Granta Publications, 12 Addison Avenue, London W11 4QR
First published in Great Britain by Granta Books, 2024

Text and illustrations copyright © Tom de Freston, 2024

Tom de Freston has asserted his moral right under
the Copyright, Designs and Patents Act, 1988,
to be identified as the author of this work.

All the poetry by Kiran Millwood Hargrave quoted in this volume was
originally published in *Orpheus and Eurydice* (Bloomsbury Academic, 2017)
and is reproduced here by kind permission of the author.

A CIP catalogue record for this book
is available from the British Library.

1 3 5 7 9 10 8 6 4 2

ISBN 978 1 78378 989 4
EISBN 978 1 78378 990 0

Typeset in Caslon by M Rules
Printed and bound by CPI Group (UK) Ltd, Croydon, CR0 4YY

www.granta.com

MIX
Paper | Supporting
responsible forestry
FSC
www.fsc.org   FSC® C171272

To Kiran

Contents

I

Splitfish

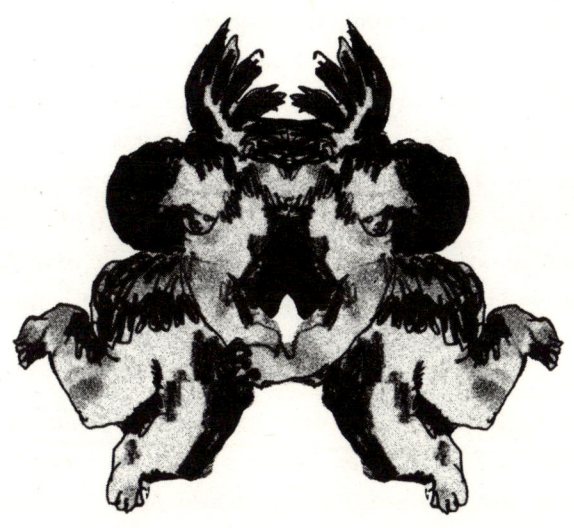

It began with a fish.

I am waiting for you. My breath fogs the windows and I repetitively smear the windscreen with my hand as I clear it, again and again. Still no sign. There's poor signal in the unit, where there's a playground right outside. It is badly designed, thoughtless.

You are in the early stages of pregnancy, and, having never been quite sure if becoming parents was something we wanted, we're joyful and excited about this new path unfolding. Worrying signs have brought us to the Early Pregnancy Unit, and partners are not allowed in due to Covid restrictions. I wait in the car park, longing to be with you, hand in hand, to feel the pulse of your fear, our fears, our hopes. It is a lesson in enforced distance.

You return. A huge smile. My lungs empty out. *It's all okay. Look. Look.* You hand me a folded piece of glossy paper, with two printed ultrasounds, one slightly more magnified than the other. A rectangle of black, framed by some tiny text, punctuated by a beam of smudged white noise. Inside a pocket of black, a curved cocoon of darkness. Inside that, two pale circles. *Twins. Those are their heartbeats. They are twins. We're having twins.*

There it is. There they are. Two fish. A split fish.

In the short ride home the future of these two lives becomes fact. We map out our future with them. As we lie in bed, curled together, you drift off to sleep and as the tone of your breathing changes, you squeeze my hand. *This is the happiest I have ever been.*

Later, still sleepless, I place my head on your belly and imagine the ocean of change churning inside your body. Imagine them there, together, swimming into form, mutating constantly. I think back to the ultrasound image and those circles. Little fish circling into life.

Here are the miraculous early stages of creation. The most everyday miracle of them. *Forms transformed to bodies new and strange.* A sacred, secular hymn of the body, of bodies, lives coming into being, *for ye have changed yourselves and all things you have changed!* And we are changed: instantly, completely.

Ultrasound images are made using sound waves. An image is made by sound, a translation from one media to another. Biomedical science is able to make the unseen internal world of the body seen. I like the word *sonography*, its feel in the mouth and ear. Fittingly melodious, right down to its dance on the page. The image is created by sound waves travelling into the body, through soft tissue, until they hit a boundary, coming to a threshold point between solid and fluid, or one density of tissue and another. These boundaries reflect back the sound waves, and this keeps happening as the computer scans different depths and densities, letting it interpret the feedback loop of sound waves and turn them into a tonal image, giving a sense of form – a two-dimensional representation of these places beyond sight.

I thought of this process as I laid my head on your belly. What was I listening for? The sonograph image itself was a song. Our twins' matter singing from within, and your body also singing. A polyphonic silent symphony.

It feels strange to say we are changed, but even in these early weeks we are. There is a new attentiveness to the world, to its details. Our lives feel achingly, overwhelmingly beautiful, almost noisy with the vibrations of possibilities. A future is unfolding in front of us, and the everyday magic of creation feels dizzying.

We recently moved house, two minutes' walk from a wood on one side and five minutes' walk from the River Thames on the other. We have done so, in large part, to start a family, for this to be the home our child or children will grow up in. There are empty spaces, waiting rooms. At the side of the house my new studio is being built, in which I'll make new artworks, and there are places in the house for us both to write in. We often collaborate, so the house will be not only for living, but working together. After over a decade in love, living a slightly itinerant lifestyle, we are ready to root ourselves and for this home to be the basis from which we grow our future together.

The pregnancy, for all its weight, is just one signifier of the life we are now trying to plot.

Next door is a burnt-out bungalow, destroyed by arson many years before. The son of the owner is a kind, interesting man, an archaeologist, and has allowed me to use it as temporary storage for my paintings. It is a black husk amid an overgrown garden. The windows are boarded up, covering shards of broken glass, sending the interior into total darkness. In one room are stacks of large, bubble-wrapped canvases, about a hundred in total, reaching the ceiling. All have been made in the twelve years of my relationship with you. Each represents a wider project, multimedia collaborations, the paintings part of broader worlds now lost. Survivors.

In a strange synergy with this burnt-out bungalow, the other rooms are full of burnt artworks, leftovers of a fire that took place in my previous studio in the garden of our old house a few months before. I lost hundreds of works. In the clear-up and house move that followed I kept huge amounts of the destroyed work. These dark rooms which now contain them are like libraries, everything carefully organised and itemised. A corner full of ash is arranged into different consistencies, from powdery residue to small shards of burnt wood. Boxes of bigger fragments, piled stacks of stretcher bars, barely a trace of canvas left on them. Buckets and cans full of thick black water scooped from the aftermath, full of smoke and debris. Shelves of paint pots, some so burnt the metal has melded, making multiple pots into one sculptural form.

In the adjoining room are a number of large canvases. Beneath the damage, the imagery of the original paintings is just about visible, although heavily deformed. In one a male figure is pulling a female figure from a blue void. The faces of both are distorted, the male face sliced through by fire. Everything is fragile and will break apart to the touch. These paintings were part of a multimedia retelling of Orpheus and Eurydice which you and I worked on a few years before, with a musician and filmmaker. The project included thirty large paintings, a short film, a collection of songs and a graphic novel threading your poems though a visual story. The project travelled as an exhibition and live performance in the years before the fire, and was an attempt to contribute to over two thousand years' worth of retellings.

Ovid recounts the story in *Metamorphoses*, his epic narrative poem chronicling the creation and history of the world through myth. In the myth, Orpheus, son of Apollo and Calliope, is a Thracian poet and musician who called Eurydice into being from a tree. Shortly after the wedding she is bitten by a snake and sinks *lifeless to the ground*: death as descent from the start. Orpheus weeps himself dry and descends to the underworld, travelling across the River Styx to find her. He hopes to *rouse the sympathy of the shades*, passing through the many corridors of death among *thin ghosts*: the selves of many lives reduced to partial forms, to traces. Orpheus meets Persephone and her husband the King of the Shades, and pleads for the return of Eurydice. Accompanying his lament with his lyre, he describes how he tried to cope but that *love was too much for me*. He suggests they might be able to *weave again Eurydice's destiny*, suggesting the return from death as a form of crafted repair. He offers up his own life if this is not possible.

They are brought to tears by his words and music and grant permission for Eurydice to follow him back to life, on the condition that he not look back until they have left the underworld, else she will be taken again. They rise up from the depths, through the silence, through the darkness, reaching towards the surface of the earth, towards the light. The description feels geological, as if the underworld is explicitly housed in the surface beneath the Thracian forest floor. Anxious that her energy might fade, he looks back. She slips away, he reaches out, he grasps, *straining to clasp her and be clasped; but the hapless man touched nothing but yielding air.* Those words, *clasping*, and *yielding air*, where the hope of a hand had been.

She falls back to death, beyond reach, her final words racing back from where her body had briefly been, fading fast and barely able to reach his ears. She returns to that same place. Orpheus is left in twice-lived grief, in which he remains locked for the rest of his earthly life. Eurydice resides forever in a double death.

Ann Wroe suggests that when Orpheus first opened his mouth, all of poetry and music fell out. From him unravelled a yet-to-happen history. What might it mean to look back at this history in reverse, in full knowledge of its entirety? Our retelling aimed to explode the previous versions, to try and build a new one. In our graphic novel and paintings Orpheus finds a minotaur in the underworld, is lost in the wrong myth. He finds monsters, horse-headed caricatures, hybrid figures, and Eurydice as a tree, sees her return to human form and then the mythic structure shifts as she resists his urge to return. He forcefully abducts her, blindfolding himself and ascending through a collage of where he had come. Agency is returned to Eurydice as at the threshold she tears the blindfold from him, forces the look, forces her return.

The final paintings were the large canvases of figures pulling each other from voids, reimaginings of Orpheus and Eurydice at the threshold between the underworld and earth, at the border-space between life and death. The figures were clearly lovers, ciphers of you and me, even bearing our resemblance. The myth space of the project had become a safe place to explore seeing you, to enter a form of an underworld we have lived in over the many years you have encountered deep suicidal depressions, each wave triggered in part by the aftershocks of a sexual assault by a stranger when we were first together in Cambridge a decade before. So those paintings were attempts to feel into what it was like to try, and maybe fail, to pull a loved one from an abyss. We had set out to open it up, until the fire closed everything back down.

But the remnants were waiting, and with knowledge of our twins thriving in the dark I felt ready for new beginnings. Of all the paths that might open up, I felt sure that one of them would be a return to the myth of Orpheus and Eurydice, and the passageways of our relationship it had illuminated. In this new house, with this new studio and your pregnancy, I was ready to find new ways in. It was now a case of waiting for the route to reveal itself. And when it came, it was not in a form I expected: I was led there by a flickering fish.

Around me, glasses clink and waiters move through the packed gallery. All of us are assembled for the opening of the National Gallery's flagship exhibition, *Titian: Love, Desire, Death*. At the bottom of a canvas, submerged in murky green water, half cut off by the painting's frame: a fish. It seems to flicker, coming into or moving out of view. I'd looked at this painting countless times, spent hours in front of its surface. Yet this was the first time I had noticed this detail.

It rises up and out of the water, into the picture plane. One perfectly circular eye wide open and glinting, mouth gaping, gasping, a flurry of daubs and dabs of paint as bubbles escape the rows of teeth, rendered as tiny dashed dots of white paint under thin, grey-green glazes. There is a loose, soft, proto-impressionistic handling of paint, a magical quality. A conjuring. Each slippery mark, each twist and turn of hand, brush and paint-covered finger on the canvas, held as if still wet, as if still mid-dash. Both form and motion seem in constant, impossible flux. The paint denies its stasis, its truth as dead matter. It is pure fish. The white highlights on a green-brown base, read in multiples as the iridescence of fish scales, the flicker of light on water and the emergence from darkness. All marks dancing, gathering into a pulsating sense of urgent life – a desperate clinging to it, or longing for, it. The edges, where fish meets water, never sharp, always dissolving, always uncertain. It is a coming into being. The passage of paint is a movement between thresholds. Paint as water, as fish, as motion, as emotion, as life. Paint as a poetic language, matter capable of transforming itself eloquently and simultaneously into multiples.

It does everything I would want paint or a painting to do. I imagine pulling a knife from my pocket, slicing out this detail and rolling it up. Maurice Sendak used to tell the story of a drawing of a Wild Thing he sent to a fan of the book. The child's mother wrote back, 'Jim loved your card so much he ate it.' Sendak said, 'That to me was one of the highest compliments I've ever received. He didn't care that it was an original Maurice Sendak drawing or anything. He saw it, he loved it, he ate it.' Perhaps I could eat this slice of Titian, this slippery fish. Love as consumption, literally all-consuming.

Someone knocks my elbow and I experience that bizarre break of focus, the pulling out of the lens. I'm back into my body. I'm hemmed in, too close to the painting, obscuring others' access. Apologising, I take a few shuffled steps back into the crowd, and the whole painting comes into view. Above the fish is a scene of violent abduction. The god Jupiter appears in the form of a wide-eyed bull, swimming upwards, while a dishevelled, terrified, wild-limbed Europa clings to his horn. The fish recedes, and the dramatic theatre of the action in Titian's *The Rape of Europa* (1559–62) takes centre-stage again.

It is the first time since the sixteenth century that Titian's suite of *Poesie* paintings have been brought back together. They had originally been commissioned in 1550 by a young Philip II of Spain, who a few years later would be king and Holy Roman Emperor. Titian, by this point already an elderly man, was given unique freedom in the plans for the scheme, which arguably was still incomplete at his death in 1576, aged ninety-eight.

The painter and the prince first met in Milan, the former brought along as part of a 500-strong party joining the prince on a grand tour across Europe, an elaborate public relations move to pave his way to power. The prince was twenty-one, the same age I was when this cycle of paintings first colonised my imagination. They next meet a couple of years later in Augsburg. Titian is the favourite painter of Philip's father, Charles V, king and emperor. Philip is keen to form an even more intimate and ambitious relationship. Over the next decade, Titian will deliver him eighteen paintings. It is an investment made in faith, in the artist over the artwork, and it is remarkable for the time to elevate the painter from artisan who fulfils his patron's vision to artist and genius. Documents suggest that the only guidance Philip gives is for the paintings to be a mythological cycle, with a series of nude women seen from different angles. The vagueness, with its focus on eroticism, would fuel the fears of Philip's advisors of his lascivious sexual appetites and liaisons.

Philip owned four copies of Ovid's *Metamorphoses*, the central source for all Titian's *Poesie* paintings. But the collection is unique in the openness of Titian's interpretations, with him looking not to illustrate moments from the poem but to translate them, to find ways of expressing the human drama that are unique to painting. The results are heralded as among the greatest achievements in Western art.

Seeing these paintings reunited in one exhibition was something I'd dreamt of for sixteen years. They'd provided me with a complete artistic language and directed me towards so many of the other painters who have guided my work. They led me to think about how poetry might be translated into paint. I was overwhelmed at the idea of seeing them all together, and arrived at the National Gallery hungry to take it all in.

They are paintings full of flesh and violent eroticism, of dramatic moments in flux. Danaë, legs apart, eyes glued to the shower of golden coins that erupt into the room. A human unable to escape her divine destiny, of rape and impregnation by a shape-shifting god. Mortal Actaeon stumbling upon Diana, goddess of hunting, and her nymphs naked at the fountain in the forest, her gaze turning him into a stag to be devoured by his own dogs. Andromeda, chained to the rocks as a punishment for her human beauty, a monster rising from the violent waves, hungry mouth wide open while, above, a gravity-defying Perseus, son of Danaë, hovers, spinning like a gymnast in the air, knife-wielding, face mirroring that of the monster he is about to kill. Venus, goddess of love and fertility, clinging with desperate desire to the beautiful hunter Adonis, her buttocks clenched as his twist and stride declare his mortal urge to hunt, and the inevitability of his grisly death.

So why, amid this tumult of drama, with this banquet of bravura paint and the unique opportunity to see these canvases together, was I constantly pulled back to this tiny fish?

On the half-drunk train ride back to Oxford from the exhibition I embark on a desperate Google search, attempting to identify the type of fish depicted in the Titian painting. As if somehow pinning the painted fish down to a particular genus might unlock iconographic or metaphorical meaning. I find the fish in a *Guardian* article about a huge collection of sixteenth-century natural history drawings and watercolours. In 2012 Florike Egmond happened upon the artworks by chance, seemingly lost, or at least forgotten, deep in the archives of the Amsterdam University Library. Among them was a delicately rendered painting of a chromis fish, its scales a shimmering array of metallic paint applied with a microscopic eye for naturalistically observed detail. It floats on cream paper, lifted from water into space, isolated to ensure a singular focus on anatomical description, on the process of identification. Painting as taxonomy.

I am convinced that this delicate watercolour is Titian's fish, lifted out of the stramash of paint and sharpened, solidified. Despite the difference in context and rendering, it has the same shape, the same peculiarly sharp triangular fin, the same profile in the mouth, eyes and gills, the same patination. Here are the details of how the fish came to be: painted in the final quarter of the sixteenth century in Venice, the exact time and place Titian painted his. Was one a copy of the other, or, more likely, was the chromis fish common to the canal waters of Venice?

We are days away from lockdown in the UK, and in Italy Covid has already turned the country into the dystopian society that will soon become a global reality. The Venetian canals, for so many years made thick with the brown sludge of the riverbed dredged up by the weight of motorboats, settle. With lockdown come clear waters, glittering emerald, a bejewelled promise of possible futures. Suddenly, the fish that populate the canals can be seen, and among them the chromis fish. As if no time had passed. We can slide between historical periods, can slip between paint and life, and find that same fish.

Titian's Venice was a city of illusions. In the waters of the canals, reflections were everywhere. Shadows lurked in the labyrinthian streets. The confluence of comings and goings, the city at the epicentre of trade and travel between east and west. Boats arriving, loaded with fabrics, pigments, jewels and stories from across the known world. In the years of Titian's life, the island of Murano, known also as the island of glass, was full of inventors and perfectors of Venetian mirrors, crafted with the same care with which Titian would craft a painting, for the same ravenous eyes of royalty, nobility and wealth. In secret spaces, gold was melded into glass as it shifted from molten liquid to thin solidifying, sparkling layers. Elsewhere, lead was used to colour the glass, turning it into a milky-white substance distributed throughout the surface, the two techniques painstakingly combined till the surface offered up a shimmering reflection.

What type of reflection was Titian's fish: a mirroring of the world or a slippery imagining? In the painting and the watercolour had I found a serendipitous rhyme between different models of the same fish, or were these reflections just further illusions, a fantasy of connection which would slip back under and disappear?

I send Florike Egmond my thoughts and she kindly and systemically outlines the differences between the chromis fish and Titian's fish, suggesting that it is perhaps not a specific fish at all but an amalgamation. The idea of a fish, fish as mutating metaphor. Suddenly all I can see is the difference between Titian's fish and the watercolour. The calm certainty of the latter. The morphing ambiguities of Titian's melding of water and fish, the sense of something shifting. Lines from the opening chapter of Ovid's *Metamorphoses* come to mind, in which chaos exploded into creation and the ordering of life:

... and lest some part might be bereft of life the gleaming waves were filled with twinkling fish; the earth was covered with wild animals; the agitated air was filled with birds.

This was it: as in the universe, so in life; as in poetry, so in paint. This passage of paint, this fish, shows the moment of mutation, the magic trick of the inanimate sticky matter layered in pulls and pushes till it finds form, and in form finds identification, and life. This was Titian's fish, not tied down to solid certainty. To Ovid again, the source of all Titian's *Poesie*, to the very first lines of *Metamorphoses*:

My soul is wrought to sing of forms transformed to
bodies new and strange!
Gods inspire my heart, for ye have changed yourselves
and all things you have changed!

This is painting. *Forms transformed ... bodies new and strange.* Not replication but creation through constant transformation. And the painter, *for ye have changed yourselves and all things you have changed!* Perhaps Titian begins with the chromis fish, but it travels in his handling. He paints not a point of destination but of departure. I look again at the close-up photos on my phone. The open mouth, the rows of gleaming teeth, the wildness of the eye possessing far more malevolence and consciousness than is usual. A monster later replicated and amplified in his painting *Perseus and Andromeda.* Wide-mouthed, wide-eyed, waiting to devour the falling Perseus.

Lockdown leads to the closure of society, and of course the Titian exhibition. Paintings which had been separated since the sixteenth century and brought back together for the public are now locked behind closed doors. It is a tiny footnote in the scheme of the pandemic's destruction, but there is something poignant about the image of the paintings alone in the empty room, museum lights off. The pandemic has been a global experience of distance. Not touching and not seeing become at points an act of love, faith and hope.

In her collection of essays *Mothers, Fathers and Others* the writer Siri Hustvedt reminds us that *Art cannot be fixed to a single location because lived experience is not left behind in the room where the object rests unseen at night after the museum has closed its doors. The art object travels in many bodies in multiple forms and it speaks and writes signs in many languages. It is a living thing.* The fish keeps swimming. It is born, or animated, in the space between the painting and the viewer. Once the encounter is over we carry it out with us, inside us. Perhaps it stays in that liminal space between being and not: coming into consciousness, requiring the viewer as a host or a magician to conjure it again inside them. Perhaps it is an act of faith. I carry the fish inside me.

The earliest painting attributed to Titian is a reimagining of the myth of Orpheus and Eurydice (*c.*1508). It is a dark painting, which for a long while was attributed to Titian's contemporary Giorgione, who would die less than two years later in his thirties. A number of Titian's early works were originally attributed to Giorgione, because of the similarity in their style at this stage of Titian's career. There is a softness to the edges of forms, contrasting with the harder-edge naturalism of Giovanni Bellini, who taught them both.

The painting is split dramatically into two narrative halves by a rock mound protruding vertically across the centre of the picture plane. In the left foreground is Eurydice in a white dress, at the moment of her first death. She is looking down towards her ankle, where a monstrous creature, all swirling, snaking, curving forms, is about to sink its deadly venom into her skin. Behind her the day holds on to the last of its light, a silhouetted tree against a distant view of Venice, moody sky tinted with the yellow glow of the sun's final throes. The landscape is an explicit metaphor for her fading light of life.

The right side of the painting depicts her second death. In the distance, a doorway into a building glows orange with the fire of the underworld, from which spills a fleeing Orpheus, head turned to Eurydice. She is positioned at the edge of the picture frame, the full force of her momentum heading inwards, towards Orpheus. But in a violent twist of her arm and shoulder is the sense of a force beyond her, triggered by his gaze, pulling her back into the oblivion beyond the frame. Back into the underworld. Her composition and perspective act as divisions of not just space, but also time.

In this first painting there is a tight, taut handling of paint, entirely at odds with the deft, silver suggestion of the fish painted at the end of his career. With that fish Titian realises the full extent of painting's poetic language, of painting's ability to shift between description, feeling and movement and to pull us up close to the surface. The fish depicts the capturing of a breath. This was what I wanted to try and do in my work: trouble the subject and pull the viewer into the picture.

Between the fish and the fire in my studio was the way forward. Their transformational power had created instability in my works. Now burnt fragments of canvas, the safe divide between the viewer and the world inside the painting was gone. Rendered sculptural by their warped materials, my paintings became objects dramatically placed within the real world. They'd entered the space of the viewer; were no longer views on to scenes but theatrical props with the viewer now an active participant. The paintings had become the bridge between realms.

I start to make paintings for you to mark the slow shifts and transformations going on inside your body. They're a mirror, a rhyme of the changes, and I want to create 280, one for each day until our babies arrive. The act of making them is like a prayer, a point of connection and contemplation, a way to speak to the babies as they circle their way into being.

I lay down paint pots on to paper, the bottoms coated in vegetable oil. Then I mix acetone with permanent marker, and pour the dark mixture around the rim. It soaks into the surface, blooms into soft-edged clouds. I have gathered bags of the ash from the burnt paintings and I sprinkle some into the liquid mixture and watch it disperse, sooty silt spreading across the page, staining and shifting.

When the paint pots are removed there are two white circles, the ink splitting and spreading like veins across the threshold. Liquid taking form, slipping from nothingness into little suggestions of life. There are tiny traces of ash crossing this border, like seeds sprayed through the air, or disrupted sediment from the bottom of a river. These paintings are my gift to you and the twins. A book of silent love songs.

Over the days and weeks, the stack of paintings in the studio is growing. New lives and possibilities growing from the wreckage of the fire, a new underworld being built from the burnt remains of a lost one. From the first sheets that are little more than empty circles, now I am trying to find forms to rhyme with the twins' developments. Inside the paired circles on the latest sheets of paper are little ink blot figures, forms floating, drifting, rhyming with each other but barely recognisable as human, barely perceptible as life.

Perhaps these circles face in multiple directions. Perhaps they are also entrances into lost pasts and myth space, portals into an underworld and also forward-facing attempts to step across the threshold between lovers. I make it my mission to build this body of paintings over the next nine months. I see them as love notes, as a form of deep connection.

We download an app showing the stages of the twins' growth. At seven weeks, it shows us, they are something closer to a sea creature, and your body is full of oestrogen and pro-gesterone. Layers of cells gathering, stitching together their hearts, knitting together a primitive circulatory system. Cells gathering as the foundations for bones and ligaments, the early architecture of bodies taking shape inside another. We feel giddy with the pace of change happening daily since the first scan, the sheer speed of growth. A new biomedical language helps us map and understand the early formation of organs, the development of eyes and ears, the buds from which limbs will sprout.

We book in for a private scan, so I can see them for myself. The studio has been my space to feel connected to them, but soon the heartbeats will be real to me as well. By now the twins will have sprouted paddle-like forms from their arm buds, then a week later this will be mirrored in their lower limbs. They will have become strange fish. Retinas will have started to form, and their brains and faces will have begun to grow. Then the first sculpting of eyes and ears, the upper lip and nose taking shape. The curved, shell-like forms blossoming, the trunk and neck straightening them out. The accelerated growth still function-ating in miniature, as they expand to about half an inch. Fingers slowly shaping, fish-like creatures slowly becoming recognisably human.

It is possible that the figures we will see in the scan have formed elbows, maybe even toes and eyelids. It is possible that the webbing between fingers and toes will have gone, that they are sea creatures in appearance no more. The scan image of the twins we see today will be a translation of two tiny, perhaps three-quarter-inch, little lives that are recognisably human. They will be becoming.

The evening before the scan I cannot sleep. Beside me, in the soft dark of the room, you are dreaming. It's sweltering, so the window is open. The cars sound like waves, the light from street lamps softens itself into the room and picks out blurred edges of things. It's a mystery what's happening inside you, right now. The soft edges of you, of them, between you both. The videos on the app are strange, intergalactic, the digitisation of the image-making unreal, using overly saturated colours. Life seems to be a process of joining and then splitting. A two-chambered heart. But also two hearts, two hopes held and growing.

The belly must feel like a huge and boundless world. The app describes them as 'your little one'. It seems weird to describe them like a possession, as if they are ours. I hope they are both their own. It says they look like a tube that is twisted back on itself. Then marries this odd poetry to the facts of their probable size and weight. *6mm 0.01 ounce.* None of this means anything to me; the information is abstract. They look more like an ear, a caterpillar, a stain of ink on paper.

Small things. What will the world seem like? It's past midnight and I'm reading some articles on my phone about what's happened in the first few weeks. They use the word 'burrow' to describe the fertilised egg implanting itself into the uterine wall. I like how active this sounds, like a seed or bulb which plants itself, which digs itself in flesh. Flesh as earth, flesh as the first home, where cells will mutate and shift and layer up to become their own flesh. They are stitching themselves into being. You are stitching them into being.

By now, apparently, they have developed fingerprints. The world will open up to them through touch. That touch will leave its trace, a little coded. Fingertips as snowflakes, patterns pressed into the surfaces of everything.

As it is still so early the sonographer does an internal scan. She is kind and patient, but it is arresting to notice how quickly the pregnant body is expected to be readily open, a site of inspection. We clasp hands, sweat gathering between us.

Our eyes are locked on the screen, on the beam of light, on the circle of darkness, in search of form and movement. Our heart rates pick up pace as we wait to hear theirs. We watch for the shifting shadows, the pulse of ink blots onscreen, expecting something akin to birds' wings, hummingbird heartbeats as you called them. A long-held breath.

There they are: question marks, arranged head to head, toe to toe. Our love is suffocating. But the atmosphere in the room shifts, at first imperceptible, but then gathers as clouds, the silence becoming a chasm.

An exhale. *I'm sorry. There are no heartbeats.*

Stasis. All those transformations absent. The unfolding futures collapsing in an instant. No more little fishes shifting into being, but rather paused, unanswered questions, descending back into darkness.

2

Step

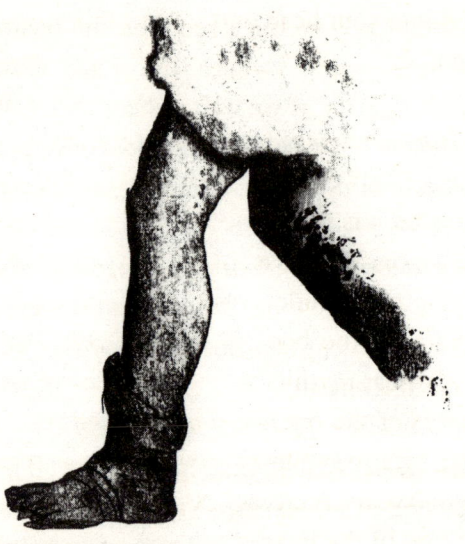

They likely wouldn't have survived birth, the sonographer said. Now they will always exist, for us, in between. Conceived a month after the fire in my studio, during the pandemic lockdown, that time of enforced distances and of non-touch, they had felt like a blessing. Now their loss engulfs everything and makes us feel as if things are breaking daily. She tells us they could not have lived long, had they been born, that the way they were tangled and tied together made them near-impossibilities, destined to end. *Better it was sooner.* It was supposed to be a comfort. We keep the scan photo from that day.

Mother. You feel as if the word has been stolen from you. Yet even in this brief window of their existence it is true, will always be true. You had recently written the first lines of a children's novel I was illustrating. One day the main character, a girl named Julia, walked into your head and started talking to you. This is what she said:

There are more secrets in the ocean than in the sky

And there she was, a child born. As Julia spoke, and as the book formed, it became clear she was a child, like all of us, with a hugely rich internal world, a world it was my task to depict.

At the centre of the book is a Greenland shark, a creature so strange it's near-mythic. A creature slowly swimming the greatest depths of the oceans, blinded by a parasite that lives on its eye in a bizarre symbiotic relationship. A creature capable of living for 800 years. A creature who seems to hold the secrets to slowing time. In the images the shark would become a metaphor, a slippery signifier of the darker spaces of the psyche. A container of things beyond itself.

The dedication in the finished book is a copy of the first painting I made of them, for them; the two circles. In the empty space of those circles there is the suggestion of deep ocean. I pinned them up in the sitting room and used them as a guide, making hundreds and hundreds of ink-on-paper paintings mimicking this space of supposed emptiness, conjuring a whole world from it, a great wide sea of works on paper covering the floor and walls of our house. I ground burnt matter and mixed it with the ink to make sharks, and birds, and lighthouses; versions of this imaginary girl Julia. But it was the sea and its depths, inspired by those paintings of them, that started manically multiplying. I imagine them both swimming forever in that ocean, in that liminal space, holding on to secrets of what could have been. A space I cannot enter.

In the book we were building a world together. The internal world of Julia was coming to life. We were making a book we hoped our children would read, creating a fictional character when the possibility of our own children had been taken from us. It was the first of your books where you'd based the main character on yourself, and it felt somehow more intimate. Later, you shared that both Julia and her mother were modelled on aspects of you: on you as a child, and you now, struggling with mental illness in your twenties and thirties. *A way of telling myself I can be sick and still be a good mum.*

I wondered if Julia provided a model for what I might do in the paintings, if I might enter the same space as you, to picture the internal landscapes of your psyche. A transgression, a space I shouldn't really access, but the desire was there. A desire to see you, to feel what you might be feeling through this loss. The ashes of the fire, the remnants of these previous worlds, felt like apt ingredients from which to construct this architecture of loss.

The hospital says you will need to take pessaries and that this will induce a miscarriage at home. *It will feel like a heavy period. It could happen within a few hours, or it could take a lot longer.* There is a casualness about the exchange, a reduction of the medicalised body to a mechanical thing. The mundanity of the instructions seems a cruelty, an erasure of the seismic nature of our grief. *At least it is early.*

You take the pessaries. We are sent home. We wait.

That afternoon I am taking part in a Zoom conversation

with the National Gallery and a tech company about Titian's *Poesie* paintings, specifically *Diana and Actaeon*. You insist I go ahead. The company are making an app to provide visitors with an augmented-reality experience of the painting, to allow the viewer to move in and around the space as if it were real.

You are lying in bed next door, waiting.

Everything was noisy, dissonant. The flat screen of my laptop, little faces in rectangles, the description of the coding, the viewer experience, the way the space of the painting had been rebuilt in a computer. I found myself expressing things I didn't think, a frictionless agreement with a set of false presumptions about the painting. And all the time, imagining.

Imagine this. Imagine a world where they had not gone. Imagine a world where I could take you all, and stand in front of the painting. Imagine a world where I could hold your hand and theirs and show you what the painting can do. I'd like to tell them just one story before they go. A story about the power of art and myth.

It begins with a poem written over two thousand years ago, by a man called Ovid. The story is one among many within a long poem full of myths about gods and humans. It is a story full of violent change, where the sacred and profane realms meet. It begins with a young man, a hunter, called Actaeon.

Actaeon, post-hunt, *strays with aimless steps through the strange wood, and enters the sacred grove* where Diana, goddess of the hunt and the forest, is bathing naked with her nymphs.

In the moments before Actaeon's arrival, the nymphs slowly and carefully lay down Diana's weapons, stripping off her clothes, tenderly bathing her body with the clear water from the fountain. Ovid describes a cave mouth dampened; the scene is charged with the eroticism of a private female space penetrated by a male presence.

The sight of Actaeon causes an immediate and visceral physical reaction from the nymphs, the whole wood filled with their sudden outcry. They shield Diana with their bodies. Diana gathers a handful of water and throws it at Actaeon, chasing it up with a threat, *tell, if you can, of what you have seen*. But words soon escape him as the sudden and dramatic transformation begins. Within a few lines of the poem he has mutated from a human into a stag. He becomes the animal he would hunt.

He runs with a speed that surprises him. In the mirrored surface of the water he sees his new animal form, opens his mouth to express horror, but no words follow. A body transformed contains the same unchanged mind. Full of fear and lost in the forest.

His dogs catch sight of him. The longest section of Ovid's poem follows, with each dog named and its key traits described. *Greedy. Savage*. Swift-footed. Trail-scented. Fierce. And finally, perhaps cruellest of all . . . *trusty*. The pack chase Actaeon across varying terrain. Actaeon flees across the same places he would have chased.

He is caught, bitten, wounded. *The whole pack gathers and they sink their teeth in his body till there is no place left to wound him*. The completeness of the damage.

Ovid describes the final flailing convulsions of a body and *a wordless head*, pained and desperate, losing its grip on life. A master torn to shreds.

The focus spins out to the sudden appearance of a crowd, Actaeon's loyal hunters, gleefully and unknowingly urging the ravenous dogs on. They call for Actaeon, worried he is missing the violent spectacle.

He might wish to see and not feel. But seeing was what got him here.

How do you translate this story from poetry into paint? How

do you translate the rhythms, the thematic concerns, the texture of language and the narrative arc into a single painted canvas? That is the conundrum that Titian took on. Ovid's poem used a rhythmic structure known as a dactylic hexameter, a poetic metre typical of many classical epics. Poems are organised by the rhythms and flow from and through lines; the equivalent in painting is the organisation of the space within the frame.

Philip II would arrive at the canvas with intimate knowledge of Ovid's telling of the story. Titian's painting is made for a private client in a private space. It is explicitly designed for a male gaze, for an intimate engagement. What is the form of the space Actaeon arrives at, that Philip confronts, that we encounter? What is the relationship between these experiences? Ovid is able to construct a collage of language, the spatial models of the poem mirroring those of the myth. A space strayed into, arrived at through *aimless steps* through a *strange wood*. To arrive at a *sacred grove, a cave mouth dampened*. A private space, a female space. How to paint this?

Titian creates a predominantly shallow space, trees and stone columns painted to form a contained enclosure into which he can organise his figures and forms. Yet there is spatial complexity and ambiguity everywhere. Through the arches, a semi-concealed view of a deep landscape and blue sky accentuates the intensity of the sacred grove. The painting is simultaneously closed and open, both inside and outside. It uniquely gives agency to the viewer, so that we are in control of the rhythm of our experience. There is no linear progression and the spatial temporal motion is conducted by the viewer.

The space of the painting doesn't hold together. It isn't meant to. If you were to build it in real space it would collapse. At various moments it returns us to the truth of the lie, a flat space in which depth is merely an illusion. We enter this unreality.

Actaeon arrives from left to right. We arrive in front of the painting, the eye going from outside to inside. We are granted a detachment not afforded to Actaeon. But in mirroring his entrance Titian creates the potential for radical empathy. Actaeon is our cipher. We move into the myth. We, all of us, are mortal figures in an immortal realm. What might we see here and what might the consequences be?

Actaeon's hips and chest are twisting, articulating the fluency of motion, which is in turn echoed by the way this has made his loose-fitting tunic rise and flow. The twists of the body are pushed just beyond anatomical limits, accentuating his movement, creating a subtle optical illusion, or better, a psychic illusion. Our minds want to correct the twist, so we are locked in a cycle in which our brains pull the hips back to what's possible and the eyes twist them back again to what we can see. We are in a loop of motion through dissonance. When we look at X-rays of the painting we see patterns similar to those in many of Titian's other paintings: a figure in constant transformation, drawn in loosely beneath the paint, limbs moved about, positions and arrangements played with and constantly evolving until the right balance and effect are found.

The word *colorito* was coined to characterise Titian and other sixteenth-century Venetian painters. It's often translated to mean colour, but, as David Rosand points out, it derives from the verb *colorare*, meaning to colour. The primary tenant of this tradition is the act of painting, of applying oil paint to canvas, a mode of painting which flourished in Venice due to the geographic and historical circumstances of its place in the trading of fabrics and pigments. For Titian and his contemporaries, painting was an evolving art, a slow build-up of figures and forms on the canvas, where change is possible at every stage. Occasionally in a Titian you will see the marks of *pentimenti*, traces of its previous existence. Flux is embedded in this painting and in the figure of Actaeon. Flux poetically expressed through the subtle contortions and manipulations of the body.

His feet give us clues. The left foot trails, weight passing on to the toes, heel lifted up, moving the body forwards, into the *sacred grove*. The right foot is placed seemingly firmly, on the point where land drops down to water. A small river flows from the central fountain, splitting the painting into two realms: the land on which Actaeon stands and the land on the other side of the river where Diana and her nymphs are gathered. The river is a boundary. Beneath his foot, the paint which describes the slope of land seems to shift, representing the decline and the movement from solidity to liquid, from certainty to uncertainty, from safety to danger. A small passage of paint and a small gradient, signifying a huge point of transition. With Actaeon's foot on this threshold, his entire existence is in mortal danger, and the changing land speaks a warning of the transmutation that awaits. On a second glance the foot shows a tentativeness, as if he'd been moving forwards but is now is doubtful and starting to shift the weight back on his heel. Regret and awareness of the danger of his *aimless step*. In that subtle rocking back, the foot shows he has *strayed* from safety.

What of our feet, what relevance here? Perhaps we stand solidly in front of the painting, taking it in, still. But we tend to move back and forth, taking in some details on the surface before moving back to take in the whole canvas, accidentally mimicking the suggested competing motions of Actaeon's body.

Then the hands. A crimson curtain hangs from a rope tied to the stone arch of the grove. One of the nymphs has pulled it back, a theatrical repeat of the reveal. Actaeon's right hand is in retreat, the arm bent, the hand held up, fingers slightly bent, a tentative stop sign. In fact, both hands are held up as if to say 'stop'. To whom? To Diana, to himself? Actaeon's left hand reaches out, forwards and into the picture plane, towards the curtain. But it floats in empty space, hovering, with the curtain just out of reach. This not-quite-touching appears time and again in Titian's paintings. Our brains want to place the hand on the surface it reaches towards. We the viewer recognise this haptic desire to touch the painting, while realising it is always beyond our reach. We sense the distance between us and not only the surface of the painting but the long-departed Titian. The painter's hands, his fingers often loaded with paint, taking over from a brush, a thumb pushing the medium into the fabric. A nail scratching into the oil to remove pigment.

Our desire to touch mirrors Actaeon's.

So, you are here, in the picture. It is no longer just what Actaeon sees, but what you see, what I see. Diana, seated, naked, on a dark-crimson cloth. The fabric is folded over the edge of the seat, draped from beneath her buttocks. It is arranged in a series of V shapes, each pleat reading as if an enlarged, repeating set of labia. Description in language makes it sound gynaecological or perversely pornographic, whereas the effect is suggestive. Paint as fabric, but fabric also gathers metaphors within its folds, sexual in association, pointing towards what can't be seen. The white highlights on the cloth now seem to glisten, the surface slick, turning inanimate matter into sex.

The folds of fabric gathered immediately beneath Diana's buttocks are also just beneath the left hand of her Black assistant. She is often called a serving maid, but it seems an overly simplistic assumption based on her role, the fact that she is clothed and her race. In contrast to the nymphs she is a riddle, and unpacking the intentions of Titian, or trying to reach clear conclusions, is tricky. A number of academics suggest, convincingly, that the trope might set her up as Diana's shadow self, and certainly there is an intimate association in their roles compared to the relationship between Diana and her nymphs. If both figures are Diana, Titian has depicted a binary based on racial grounds. She certainly, however, seems afforded agency and potency. She is too palpably flesh and blood to be a mere signifier of Diana's psyche.

Look back to her left hand and the way the thumb seems to be softly brushing the pink pleats, to the three fully bent fingers, to the half-bent forefinger. The hand, hovering just at the edge, just above the fabric, is in the motion of pleasuring. So often, in paintings such as the *Venus of Urbino* (1538) or the Prado version of *Danaë* (c.1560s), female hands are positioned in fabric or between legs with fingers bent, as if masturbating. In *Danaë*, another of the *Poesie*, a blurred-out hand between the legs seems to be opening her up for the shower of golden coins that Zeus has transformed into. The body is depicted as a supplicant slot machine, a surreal, ambivalent, perverse depiction of a scene of sexual abduction.

She exists at the edge of the painting, her body outside the frame, as if in transition and between worlds. In paintings the margins are never places to be ignored. Here she is, draped in beautiful clothes, painted with deep attention. In Patience Agbabi's poem 'About Face' (2012), written in response to this painting, the sewing maid is given voice: *you should have looked at me*. Agbabi brings her alive, feels into the figure, all the action and drama viewed from her viewpoint. Agbabi unfolds her inner psychological working, from the erotic suggestion of the thumb on the fabric through to the movements of the body and the expressions of the face. A character full of her own desires and appetites. A reminder, should one be needed, that desire does not just work in one direction. The lyric eye of the poem shifts the gaze from Actaeon to Diana, meaning the sight, the insight and the desire becomes hers, and therefore the power.

Beside her, Diana's pose is an awkward one, shifting from a reclining position to upright. The whole body is an arrangement of twists and counter twists. It is what would be labelled *contraposto*, which literally translates to mean 'opposite'. It is a device often used in classical and Renaissance sculpture and painting, where one part of the body is weighted or twisted in one direction to allow the other to move in opposition. Here the function is not merely beauty: it is dramatic. As with Actaeon, Diana's anatomical impossibilities are not inaccuracies but ways in which to articulate a pulsing moment in dramatic flux. Her body acts, as with many of Titian's bodies, like a proto version of the shower scene in Hitchcock's *Psycho*. There, the actual meeting of knife and body is never shown, but rather, through the repeat flashing between moments we fill in the gaps, creating the motion and impact of the violence. Here Diana's body was clearly, just a moment ago, in a state of total exposure. Her left foot is still being cleaned carefully by her nymph, toes splayed in delight. Her legs are in the act of closing. The toe of her right foot dips into the river, crossing the divide that Actaeon's feet sit behind.

The foot moving from the dry land, the toe dipping suggestively into the wetness of the water, the calm certainty of the entrance, a move of both power and bliss. The reflection of the foot in the water, an image of the body melting and dissolving. Her entire body speaks of her interrupted pleasure, not for Actaeon, Philip II or us. It's a painting of female pleasure, not male, which it holds purposefully beyond us, tantalisingly out of reach.

The five nymphs, all naked, are positioned in the space between Diana and Actaeon. Their nudity is amplified by Actaeon and Diana's clothed attendants. Each figure is seen from a different angle, each in a distinct pose. Collectively they fulfil one of Philip's requirements: that the *Poesie* paintings show various naked women from a variety of angles; but each figure demonstrates Titian's ability to turn oil paint into flesh. White built up, thin layers of colour pulled through and laid over. It's a slow process, the paint not just contouring the shape of the body but slowly and surely forming it. Pushing at the edges, carefully mapping the way light falls across an area of flesh. The paint never feels flat or solid: there is always softness and variety.

The painting itself is a body, or a metaphor of the body; the canvas a skin stretched across a wooden skeleton. And alongside flesh are a cacophony of surfaces, of different forms of materiality rendered in paint: fur, glass, stone, water. Paint is a trickster always able to be something else. A painting as a make-believe space which confesses its artifice. Paint declares itself as pigment suspended in a medium layered over a canvas, but also all these other things at once. A painting which never tries to claim it is real life. We are always aware of the construction. The magic happens in the shift between states.

This magic seems absent, entirely, from the augmented virtual-reality model of Titian's *Diana and Actaeon* I am being shown on the Zoom call. I'm distracted by the idea of your growing pain, by the slow onset of the miscarriage. Your mother is with you, but I feel a deep guilt at the distance between us. Why am I here, not there?

In this poem translated into paint, I am reminded of language being your domain, and paint being mine. I think back to your poems from our Orpheus and Eurydice project, to the printed-out versions which had been burnt in the fire, now stacked in a box next door. Of the type of female spaces they articulate, of what it might mean to enter or translate these. I think of you next door, being made animal by pain.

I hear you shift quietly from the bedroom to the bathroom.

Then deep moans, crying, the calling of my name. It's embarrassing how slow and awkward I am in my attempts to extricate myself from the call. You are hunched on the toilet, and when I enter, your eyes are bright with panic. *They said there wouldn't be pain. Make it stop.* You seem elsewhere, vanished inside your body, consumed entirely by what it is doing to you, by what their passing is doing to you. The body sent, artificially, into the convulsions of a labour, the muscular contractions of something like a birth. I am utter inadequacy. I run a bath, lift you in.

There is a long blur of pain that seems to mount, and suddenly there they are. A small pink form floating among blood, drifting alongside you. The starts of them. We hold each other, and then you scoop the sac into your hands. You climb out, gently wash it under the tap, cleaning off the excess blood. What remains sits in the palm of your hand. Intact. You run two fingers across the seemingly opaque surface, the gentlest of touches, a caress.

I remember being in this same bathroom when the worst nearly happened, when the grip of your depression had become suffocating, when to not exist had seemed the only logical option. But here, in this moment, you are teaching me to see in the dark. You hold them both, whatever they both now were, in your palm. You are looking with such care and attention, with an intensity of love and curiosity. I see you are not afraid to look, or to see the beauty that is here. Here, in what is left of them, the miraculous and the terrible meet. The miracle of what was, of what could have been, held forever in this moment. *They're just like the images on the app*, you say. Forming into something human, like the early stages of a painting, form emerging from matter. Their minuscule bodies, little paddle limbs. Eyes, lidless. Together, never alone. Your touch, with its impossible smallness, makes me realise your capacity to love. What a tender mother you would have been to them.

We make a small fire, for a small ceremony. We carefully lay them on the tiny pyre, strike a match and watch in silence. We load the ashes into a glass jam jar. You separate out a small amount for your mother to scatter in her garden. I remain mute, unable to gather the words or breath to make sense of the dissonance I feel at this splitting of them. As if, somehow, it was to separate them, an act of spiritual cruelty. I know it's ludicrous, but the feeling is choking me from within. Later I tell you, and rather than relief I feel I've poured the same feelings into you, polluting what had been an act of love with my irrational pain.

I've been struggling to paint. To know how or what to paint, let alone why. Paint, or painting, has been my access point to the world, to feeling into it, to thinking through it, to understanding my relationship with it. But now the world is this: grief. Future possibilities taken. Waiting. Distance.

Maybe what I will paint is this in-between world. I want to open up the language of paint, to start again, to throw out what I have done. I want to enter the body and enter the gaps between us.

> *My soul is wrought to sing of forms transformed to*
> *bodies new and strange!*
> *Gods inspire my heart, for ye have changed yourselves*
> *and all things you have changed!*

Bodies new and strange. Forms transformed, transforming. I want to capture this changing, morphing matter in paint, the poetry of possibilities. And I don't yet know what this means, let alone looks like. I have a desire to express beauty, in its wonder and terror. A desire to let go of design and be led by the work; to let it unfold as a form of creation itself. Mapping our experiences as they unfold is an exercise in hope.

In a note on my phone I see a typo. Where I meant to write blind faith I wrote blind father. Perhaps I am holding on to the hope or memory of being a father. Like Actaeon, the figure who enters the female space, I'm a stranger here, trespassing. Entrance itself is a form of violent transgression. I will only ever be at the threshold looking in, as Orpheus stands at the threshold of the underworld. The stakes are high and I can feel the threat of transformation beyond my control. Yet I can't be merely a static witness. Even as the twins have gone, I want to take them with me on that journey.

3

Breath

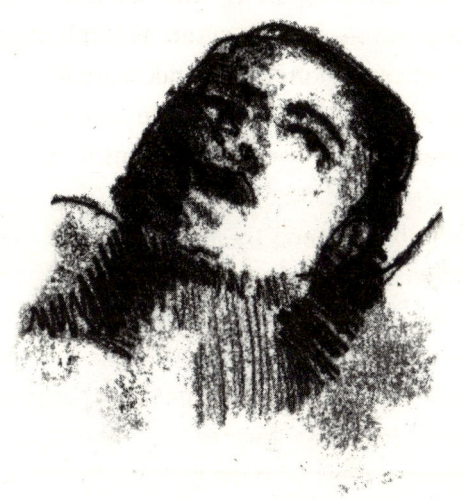

When they gave us the final scan there were two images. The sonographer handed us the thin printout folded at the seam, presuming we would not want to see it. Now it is smoothed flat by repeated looking, but the folding caught my attention.

The old English root of the verb *fold* has, suitably, a double meaning. To *become doubled upon itself* and, referring to the body, to *give way*, or *fail*. Embryological development is one of enfolding and unfolding. In the fourth week the forming body folds inwards, head and tailbone curled towards each other. Drawing in on itself, the emergent body is like a shell or fossilised sea creature. Then, slowly, an unfolding. The stretching of the spine and back, the settling into a recognisably human form. Beyond a mirroring of the biological developments, this folding felt true to the psychological experience of the hope we held for them and the loss that followed.

In the few weeks of their existence, everything changed. Time is an accordion opening then closing. They taught us about the quantum mechanics of self. We split, daily, like mycelium. Whole other versions of self and possible selves rolled out ghost futures, shadow histories, parallel existences. They were hovering in the space of coming into being.

I see them, and the other us, living a life different to ours. I see two mouths learning to shape sound in meaning. I see stuttering steps. I see tired eyes. I see them not as what would-have-beens but as things existing in another version of the universe. It makes me dizzy, it makes me joyous, to think of those versions amongst the infinite mass, amongst the daily proliferation of new paths. I see this version so clearly, and let it sit, faded, glowing, distant on the horizon. In moments there are cracks in the space-time continuum, or it is merely the hope our brains wire us into, a mirage. Conjured or real, these moments I glimpse are filled with joy, melancholy, hope and grief.

In the months they grew, those weeks before they were no longer, I'd sit by the river in Oxford while you and our best friend, also newly pregnant, slid into the river and swam. Two bodies melting into the brackish water, beneath the dark-green reflective surface, ripples drifting out and back to the river edge. I'd think of the twins in the dark underwater cave of your body. I have a photo of you emerging from the river, small in the near-distance, blurry and exuding contentment. They pivoted how I saw the world. They brought my inattention back to the present and to the marvels around us. In Norfolk, I sat on the beach holding two pebbles in my hand as you walked slowly into the long shallows of the sea, until you were deep enough to swim. The sudden appearance of a seal alongside you, a kindred being. I felt sheer astonishment at the two pebbles: how they came to be, the time over which the water massaged them and sculpted them into smoothness. Holding these for them, till we could hold them in our arms.

We took their jam jar ashes with us in my coat pocket, searching for the moment to let go. We went back to the same patch of beach in Norfolk, and you walked back out to the same and different sea. You are not ready to let them go, neither of us are. We drink a large bottle of our favourite dark Norfolk ale and watch the sun slide slowly across the wide horizon.

We see them everywhere. In a fallen conker from the twin horse chestnut trees outside our house, opening its prickly skin to reveal two perfect forms nestled inside. A few weeks after we move in we discover that one of the trees is sick and will need to come down. When it is felled and sliced into rounds the tree repeats itself, one slice folding out the mirror of its neighbour. Then they are in Tuscany, a double rainbow curving across the hills of Orciatico. I catch them in the in-between spaces, when I am sleepless in earliest morning, creeping around a dark house, the glow of the street lights scattering shadows of the shutters across the floor. I sit with them till the blue of the morning starts to rise from the orange glow. Ghosts in the gloaming of the day. In Venice, in the flickering water spaces. I see them everywhere. In Wales, on a pebbled beach in two stones with matched quartz bands. On a research trip to Paris, curled in the slice of an orange. The thin translucence, the sunset glow. They are in the dried lavender and rosemary on my desk. I see them often in the faces of other babies. I am glad they were never, and will never, be alone.

*

On the wall of Erin Lawlor's studio, next to a recent canvas, is a small printout of *Perseus and Andromeda* (*c*.1554–6), one of Titian's *Poesie* paintings. Andromeda is chained, head turned, red slashes of her parted lips emerging from the dark; the sea monster, writhing violently out of the waves, teeth bared, is ready to devour Perseus. Perseus, upside down in a gymnastic defiance of gravity, is about to fall, either to his death or victory into the churn of sea and the monster's mouth below.

In the twists and folds of the waves, the translucent scraps of fabric around Andromeda and the clothes swirling around Perseus are expressions of held breath. Paint pauses motion, stills time. The wild cacophony of what can be held in paint marks. Erin Lawlor's paintings are a radical reimagining of these moments, amplifications of an exhaled breath. They are abstract fights against death.

Lawlor arrived at paint through a frustration with the limits of language. She was a writer hemmed in by the certainty that language demanded. Language, in its precision, couldn't get at feeling in the way that paint could. Following the suicide of her brother she began painting portraits. In the following year her father was diagnosed with thymoma, and the recurrence and progression of the cancer over the next decade coincided with her continued drive to capture likeness in paint. While her ex-husband was at work reconstructing the faces of patients at his surgery, she was at home reconstructing his face and their child's in paint, as if by capturing their image she could keep them alive. She fought the inevitability of transience and mortality through paint. Following her father's death she continued down this path for another year, before she realised she had painted herself into a dead end, and then turned towards abstraction as an antidote.

She has developed an artistic language of evolving richness.

Paintings are made on stretched canvases laid down on her studio floor with a protective sheet beneath to capture the marks and spills that transgress the edges. Edges which Lawlor often photographs and posts on social media, reminders of the physicality of the paintings. The edges reveal secrets. She also posts photographs of the grids of sunlight which stream through the studio wall and pattern themselves across the surfaces of the painting. Although informal, these photographs draw our attention to the materiality of the surface of her paintings, situating them in the real – not digital – world.

Alongside the canvases are trays of pre-prepared paint, oils diluted with solvents and mediums. Wide, flat brushes are loaded up, paint is pulled across the surface, the mark of the brush is made and at points dissolves when wet paint meets wet paint. Lawlor is interested in how paint is applied into marks that encode mutated memories of its formation. The brush is manoeuvred by the turn of a hand, the twist of an arm or the dynamic shift of an entire body through space.

In our chats Lawlor draws a direct comparison between the making of a painting and the operating theatre. The painter is a surgeon, perhaps even a midwife; the painting a body. For Lawlor, theatricality is important. The solvents she uses mean she operates in a limited window of time, pressure forcing a heightened engagement with looking, thinking and mark-making. She says she wants to *leave everything there, all of yourself.* The surfaces and resulting canvases are the product of an emptying out of self, and even after Lawlor has stepped away she leaves a deep imprint. Her paintings are poetic assertions of existence, a resounding cry of *I was here*, made potent by her absence when the viewer arrives and becomes the primary agent. The paintings might be abstract, free of explicit imagery or figuration, but body and breath pulse through them.

Much of the literature about Lawlor's work describes it as Baroque. The term was coined in the nineteenth century as a catch-all word for a historical period and a genre of art and literature, unified by its excesses, stylistic inventions, exaggerations and embellishments. Applying this term to a contemporary painter is a historical anachronism, but her work does capture a Baroque sensibility, a tendency towards similar stylistic distortions, articulated in a contemporary visual language.

The Baroque is most purely expressed in her fascination with folds. The surfaces of her paintings are records of the actual folding of one motion or medium into another, and then the subsequent surfaces which create the illusion of folding forms. Baroque artworks are full of fabric as expressions of excessive distortions, showing how it might vanish into or emerge from itself. In the looping depths of Baroque folds are infinite possibilities, sudden cancellations, a constant movement between creation and erasure. In Lawlor's paintings, folds are abstract, free of a context. Spatial illusions take on complex explorations of scale, shifting fluidly from micro and macro, while constantly returning us to the trick: the gathering of the paint on the surface, the flatness of the canvas.

Lawlor's painting captures a paradox of two-foldness, in its relationship between surface imagery and the illusion of depth. She cites Pier Kirkerby's painting and writing as a direct influence on her work. His texts speak openly about the *fundamental dishonesty of painting*. Lawlor's partner is a book maker, and few can know more about the secrets, lies and truths that can be held in folds than bookbinders. Of the many reasons why physical books have survived the digital age, one must be the act of opening, turning and closing these enfolded pages. There is magic in that act of unfolding: an act of faith, a joint belief between writer and reader in the leaps of imagination we are all capable of.

The word 'Baroque' originally referred to a naturally formed type of irregularly shaped pearl. At the bottom left of Titian's *Perseus and Andromeda*, on the rocks beneath Andromeda's feet, are two open shells spat up by the waves. Lift them to your ears, hear the sea. Dive in beneath the surface and find more shells, closed and holding secrets. Inside and hidden, a slow process is taking place, layer by layer, concentric circles of calcifying matter shaping into a pearl. A mutation occurs and rather than being worked towards a perfect white sphere the matter gathers into a strange, undefinable shape, its surface not milky-white but an iridescent galaxy in miniature. Eventually the shell will unclasp and reveal its creation as an accidental gift. Grasp it in your palm, swim up to the surface, take in a breath. Keep swimming, back to land, then open your fist. Picture the peculiar pearl. Hold on to it.

During the Covid pandemic, Lawlor was diagnosed with a rare form of lung cancer, which she believes was triggered by stress and grief, and possibly cross-generational trauma, her body bearing the brunt of psychological damage. She'd previously experienced a late-term miscarriage. The exact medical causation of cancer seems, in this context, less important that the correlation made and felt by the patient.

On Instagram, Lawlor posted a photograph taken on the day of her lobectomy. An arrow is drawn in clear black marker pen on her left shoulder, pointing down to the site of her damaged lung, to ensure the correct one is removed. *Deep breath, ready to go under.*

All cells reproduce, but cancer is the presence of aberrant growth; mutating and spreading. Some of the literature I had been reading seems to discuss cancer as something that happens to the body, like a colonisation or controlled growth taking over the machinery. Yet a friend who is a consultant oncologist corrects my assertions, reminds me that *cancer is part of the body; it is the body.*

Viewed through an X-ray, our lungs look like the root systems of a tree. Great networks of fibres, knitted together to create a diaphanous bag, contracting and expanding as waves of air are pulled into our chests, filtering out the oxygen to transport around our body. There is something of the deep ocean about the body's interior, and going under for surgery can feel like descending to the darkest, deepest depths of that ocean.

The Mariana Trench, in the Pacific Ocean, is the world's deepest oceanic trench, at over 36,000 feet. On a recent descent an explorer saw a plastic bag floating about like some kind of lifeless, man-made jellyfish, another contribution to the growing mass of single-use plastic in the ocean. In a post-human landscape, the Anthropocene will have left its own strata in any geological cross section, a multicoloured conglomeration of plastic pollution, a dulled rainbow speaking of the damage wrought. These same microplastics are found in our bodies, breathed in, ingested, travelling to our organs through our blood, lodged in the deepest depths of our lungs. The latest scientific research hypothesises a direct link between this proliferation and lung cancer, the plastics seen as potential instigators of cellular transformation. We fill the air with these invisible pollutants, then with each breath taken in we sow the microscopic seeds of future illness.

In the agonising, lengthy period between Lawlor's diagnosis in mid-July 2021 and her operation at the end of September, her creative output increased in urgency. In a message she sends me on Instagram she calls it a *window of work*. It's a poetic phrase: the work as a view into, or out of something. The self, the body, life? Her daughter joined her in her work, *doing heavy lifting but also just talking, listening. Putting things in place in case, teaching her the studio workings, the database.* An intense preparation for the possibility of death, she prepared paintings which might end up speaking posthumously. She tells me, *it felt so important that it be very alive, and positive.* She cites Joan Mitchell: *painting is the opposite of death.* Later I google the quote and am intrigued by how it extends beyond the iconic aphorism. Mitchell continued, *it permits one to survive, it also permits one to live.* The paintings in this period of waiting are assertions of life.

There has always been beauty in Lawlor's work, but it is unleashed in the large canvases she made during this period. They are a dance, a *wild celebration abasing death*, as Lawlor puts it. She cites Peggy Lee's song *if that's all there is … let's keep dancing*, and its defiance in the face of nihilism. She makes a connection between her aims and Titian's late work, to paintings such as *The Flaying of Marsyas*, where the surfaces of the canvases become more open, the marks more expressive. Faced with mortality, these paintings are engagements with the fragilities of the body.

In the triptych *La Vie en Rose* (2021) we are waltzed into beauty, before being spun into a frenzy. It is a musical painting. Each canvas is 190x130cm, roughly human-sized, or perhaps the size of a coffin. Spaces to live in, spaces to die in. Pinks, reds and blues dance among deep dark-grey and brown swirls. We are pulled on to, into and back out of the space of the paintings in a motion of a musical maelstrom that seems to gather speed, becoming almost breathless. The title is a reference to Edith Piaf's post-war hit, a song of love and life in the aftermath of so much loss. The title is usually translated as an idiom – life seen in rosy hues – but it translates literally as life in pink. Her painting takes us there. Life is beautiful. Life is to be embraced, like painting, for the intensity of the now.

In *Summer Storm* we are confronted by a diptych dominated

by reds, crimsons and light pinks, with flashes of grey, yellow and blue. Colour is liberated, and there is a boldness and looseness to the marks as they fold over, out of and back into each other. The diptych form exaggerates the similarities and differences in each canvas. Either elaborate and intricate panel could morph into the other. An inhale and exhale, two sides of the same mirror, opened out to be viewed at once. Light and joy are unleashed, but unsettling darkness too. Folds conceal more than they reveal. The viewer hovers in a space between light and shade, the known and unknown.

Lawlor was taken aback by her response to the removal of her lung. She says, *I was surprised that the overriding sense re my lung was gratitude. I felt it had taken layers of grief over the years for me.* She felt a gratitude for the lung's ability to take air in and to let air out. To facilitate not just physical survival but psychological survival. Breath by breath.

Among the large bombastic canvases are two small paintings, *Souffle I* and *Souffle II*, the French word for breath. After the shows and sales that followed the creation of this body of work, she decided to keep hold of these two small canvases. In their intimacy of scale and mark, they resonate at a different frequency to the large multi-panelled paintings. Both are 60x45cm, about the size of a screen on which an oncologist might view biomedical images of the body. The size of our chests. The movement of the marks is slower, isolating our attention to this space and to the motion of the hand. They are deliberate and elongated. They are dark paintings, dominated by nearly black and grey, though in *Souffle I* a burst of red flashes against the dominance of monochrome. Looking closer, more red below, and green. The greys pulled over, through and into the colour, the vibrant dragged brush marks of paint full of air. In *Souffle II* colour is almost entirely absent, mere flickers between and beneath marks. It reminds me of rain clouds in a late work by John Constable. The vertical drags of paint across the surface in the Constable are perfect articulations of the way rain can sheet down. And from Constable to Keats's 'Ode on Melancholy':

> *But when the melancholy fit shall fall*
> *Sudden from heaven like a weeping cloud*

Lawlor and Constable catch this suddenness, of melancholy as a cloud emptying itself. But there is a different kind of verticality to Lawlor's work that reaches for the poetic depths of Keats, beyond the meteorological depths of Constable. Lawlor makes marks when the paintings are laid flat, and then we view the canvas hung on the wall. This shift from the horizontal to the vertical enacts the kind of drama of Keats's sudden rainfall. They seem to hover in a moment of extreme tension. The paintings themselves as a pair of lungs, as sites of breath. A breath in, a breath out, a motion and movement with the fear and threat of collapse, and stasis.

Meaning is secondary here. The central relationship between the viewer and the paintings is one of feeling. Our visual engagement is a route into our feelings about the world and about ourselves. The estranged marks left by the brush are signifiers and stimulators, of feeling within us. It is an intimate exchange, akin to love. In a world of instantly digestible and scrollable images, these canvases offer small moments of connection to the materiality of the world.

Lawlor says of these works, *It really did feel like a conversation with my lung, gratitude and a homage as I was preparing to let it go.* She notes the strange synchronicity that her lung was removed on the same day her brother took his life years before, the autumn equinox. It is autumn equinox again when we have this exchange.

There are intimate bonds between a painter and the painting, just as there are between lovers. In the intensity of this intimacy, I have been guilty of collapsing the gap both in my paintings and in my relationship with you. In my paintings, presuming they are subservient products of my imagination. Ignoring the life present in them and the exchange outside my control. In the weeks and months after the loss of the twins I had been so focused on the *you* of them that I had allied the two that made the we or us into a singular. In our hope, in our loss, in our grief, I had collapsed the separation between us as individuals.

There was a huge distance from me to the twins, these folding and unfolding forms inside your body. I felt a grief about this distance; their lives were beyond me, in every sense. For you, it was the opposite. There was no separation between you and them. Foetal cells and DNA have been shown to stay in the mother's body for decades after birth. The exchange of matter, and of support, works in both directions. The twins were forming from you, not just in you, both growing and changing together.

Each week prior to the discovery of our loss, you would show me on an app how the twins were developing. I remember you telling me about the development of their lungs. At five weeks the lung would appear as a bud-like form, branched out from a tube-like collection of cells. We marvelled at the way that in the very moment we were talking about it this bud would have been splitting into two and folding out. You read somewhere that the twins would soon be mimicking breathing, in preparation for its possibility. It seems they were permanently paused around the seven-week mark, just as the lungs began their second stage of development.

When you showed me the images and read me the texts they sounded like poems, or perhaps that's just the way words taste in your mouth. There is a kind of lyricism unique to science, in the magic of a fact explained. To say that the lungs were developing *tree-like structures* paints a picture of a forest growing inside you, the inside of the body a site of Ovidian transformation. We watched animations of how the lungs would divide and divide, fractals folding out over and over like the branches of a tree. I marvelled at how your breath was theirs, transported through your blood to them.

The connection between you and the twins manifested itself in your desire to keep hold of the ashes. We had various plans for where we might scatter them, so took them travelling with us. Into forests, to rivers, to the sea, to cliff edges. To places full of old memories, and new places which might hold only the memory of them. We searched the garden, thought of planting flowers or trees under which they could be scattered. Yet they kept coming home with us, in the little glass jam jar, back into the little wooden box you had made.

We take them to Wales to search out a spot to send them to the sea, packed carefully in my rucksack. We wander down to Rhossili Bay beach, the remains of the *Helvetia*, shipwrecked in 1887, the only thing punctuating the golden glow of the sand. As the tide works its way outwards the carcass is revealed. We walk out to meet the edge of the sea, wander the strange skeleton of the ship. We look across the sea to Worms Head in the distance, decide that that is where we will let them go.

We wait for the tide to go out, drop down the cliff-edge path to the exposed, slippery rocks at the start of the climb. It feels like a pilgrimage. We rest at the point where the cliffs open up to views across rocky bays, full of seals inelegantly splayed across the rocks, in such contrast to their extraordinary grace when they slip back into the water. We think it is a sign, as you feel connected to seals, you think of yourself as a selkie, happiest and most in your body in water.

We clamber onwards for another hour or two until we reach the end point, with the view out to the wide sea crashing on all sides. We walk to the edge, lean over. The sea is foaming as it meets the rocks, like a thousand hands reaching up and beckoning us down. I kick a piece of grit over the edge, and it seems to drift in the wind rather than plummet, an endless fall down to the waves below, vanishing out of sight. You cannot do it, cannot let them go here. *It feels too like oblivion.*

I had been thinking about how Erin Lawlor's work related to my own painting practice, but her canvases also revealed something about our intimate relationship. The pair of *Souffle* paintings were devised by Lawlor not as a diptych but as two connected independent paintings. They were, in that sense, like the twins. But they were also paintings of desire. It is a strange, dangerous thing to say, but I desire your grief. I desire to feel what you feel, to have that depth of connection. I'd like to imagine that my desire is to relieve you of it, so I can consume it for you. But that is not all. I am jealous of your grief and of the unbreakable connection that you had, have, for our twins. This grief, the twins, you will always be just beyond my reach.

What am I painting? I don't know. All this loss has made me want to start over. I know I am setting out to make paintings of you, for you. I know you are my subject. But I don't want to make portraits in the conventional sense. I don't even know if I want to make paintings with images, figures or narrative, let alone with a premeditated design or content. I am in a process of exploration, trying to find a language that might do justice to how it is to be in love with you, to desire you, to see the wonder and complexity of you. To see your joys, your suffering, your body. I desire to enter you, in every sense.

The etymology of empathy means to enter someone. My desire for empathy, when it comes to you, is all-consuming. Love is devastatingly greedy. My desire is physical, active. It is fuelled by sexual desire more than bodily lust. I have a desire to climb inside the other, the lover, fully. The urge feels dangerous in the way it slides into possessiveness, into a desire to totally devour, to totally know. Fold after fold after fold. There is a libidinal quality to the connections I wish to make, from feeling to flesh. A strange complexity emerges from my sexual appetite and this conflicted objectification. I am the root of the pregnancy from which the loss came. The seed of it. I feel a deep and ridiculous guilt.

The limits of the stretched canvas bother me. The rectangular frame, the edge, the contained and circumscribed image. It felt, suddenly, murderous of possibilities. So I start making folded paintings. I work on unstretched and unprimed rolls of canvas, large as cathedral doors. I work on them during this period of loss, over months. I pour, spray and chuck buckets of paint, varnishes and turpentine at the surface. I lay whole rolls out across the garden of our new house, long grass growing around the fringes. Paint pools into puddles, runs like rivers into the grass and earth, soaks the grey concrete slabs of our patio. When the rain comes I let it gather across the surfaces. When the sun arrives it accelerates the speed of the paint drying, leading to cracks and splits of paint all over. I keep adding to the soup, to the mixture, like a spell for who knows what? Sometimes I turn the rolls of canvas over, so there is no front or back, merely two options for the same experiment. I become more interested in the marks that happen on the underside, in the ones that are further distanced from my knowledge or control, the ones

I cannot see so have to imagine. Sometimes the weight of the canvas pushes the surface down firmly into the long grass, lets it print itself on to the canvas courtesy of the wet paint.

At various intervals I fold the paintings. Sometimes the folds are straight, splitting the ten-metre length in half, then in half again, to leave large, folded squares. At other times I will fold at an angle, and keep going until the canvas will bend no more. After each folding I walk along the crease to flatten it, paint squelching where it gathers at the seams, pouring out at the edges. I lift heavy slabs of concrete and lay them on top to weight it down, keep going till there is a metre-high stack of concrete slabs on top. The painting is now pressed between land and concrete, pressed against itself, imprinting on to itself. A painting recording, making, unmaking itself. Things will happen here I can't control, a process involving time, weather, weight and the materiality of the hodgepodge of ingredients that have been added, both consciously and accidentally, to the concoction. Colonies of ants appear from beneath the painting. Snails gather.

When the Orpheus of our graphic novel steps into the underworld it is a folded space. Each door leads him into a closed-off place, bent back on itself. The architecture of the underworld is one of enclosed memory. All the versions of the myth over 2,000 years of retellings are echoing through the underworld. He walks across a folded map, searching for a way in. The geography he is used to doesn't work here. Perhaps these folded paintings are – if not excavations of an underworld – connected to the formation of one. They are an attempt to construct entrances into it.

We are ready to start trying for a child again. I am not sure what to say, or why to say it, or even whether words might be the right thing to offer up. I want to show you what I was seeing in you, what I was feeling or failing to feel, why when we were grieving I needed to be in the garden folding huge canvases covered in pools of paint. I want to use words to say: here, this is what I was thinking. This is an apology. Or maybe this is language as a recovery of a memory. I seemed to be so dulled of feeling when you were so full of it. Language as matter, slick sticky matter; language as paint. I am using your medium, words, when mine seems to fail. Making a text as a hand which reaches out to yours, which brings you in, next to me. I want to close that gap between us, or to enter it unbodied, together, you and me. Or perhaps I am writing about failures. The failures of paint and words. If I can create something, some kind of life, from paint or words, I hope it will act, impossibly, as a conduit to the life we are trying to create together.

We had been holding our breath, had plummeted deep into an internal ocean. These paintings were an attempt to rise up, to catch the air again, to turn it into breath.

4

Hatch

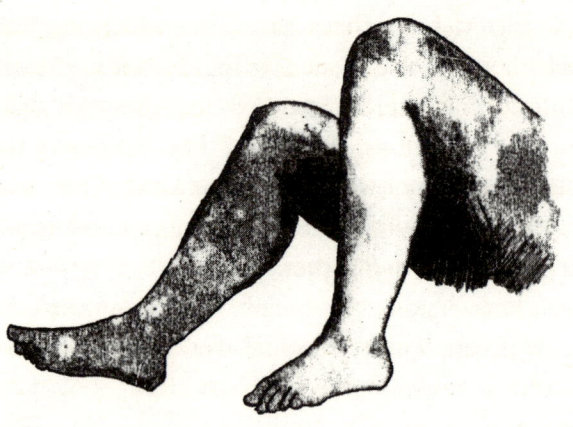

We are fixed in a pattern of trying, calendars structured around ovulation cycles. Then the waiting, the hope there is a meeting inside you, gestation starting. We read more and more about the biology of conception, as some kind of prayer, as if to read about how it happens might will it into being. We focus on the pleasure of trying, not wanting this act to become purely functional. It feels more important than ever that in this period of backwards-facing grief and forward-facing fear we maintain the immediacy and connection of that intimacy. Yet there is still a need to think through timings, or you lifting your legs after sex, stretched up the wall.

As we wait for the earliest chance to test we talk to your

belly, to that cluster of cells, praying without any formal faith that they have become a blastocyst, made by cells constantly dividing into halves, one of which will become the placenta and one the embryo. Another article describes it as a *hollow ball of cells*, yet there seems nothing hollow about it. These rapidly dividing cells, accelerating towards existence, carry the weight of possible life.

It is strange to know that what we are waiting for – an arrival and attachment – won't be seen or felt. The blastocyst will arrive in the uterus and implant into the endometrium. The official term for this is hatching, where the outer layer of cells is shed and the outer layer of the blastocyst knit themselves into the outer layer of the endometrium. A protein described as 'sticky' will be released to bind these two layers together. To bind, to stick, to attach.

The two-week wait passes and the day to test arrives. You pee on a stick, long minutes of our lives. Only one red line, not pregnant. You try the next day, hoping you had tested too early.

No line. We lie silently together, my lips pressed to your forehead. I take the test to the bin, and there, I am sure, is the faintest of lines. We look again, and over the coming minutes it gets darker. The next day we test again, and the next, and each day it gets stronger. You are pregnant.

We know we should remain detached and keep a rational distance. We are no longer naïve to the high risks of loss so early in a pregnancy. Yet our attachment is not contained. I think of that word hatching, pray that the splitting and clinging continues. We now wait and give ourselves over to the hidden act of creation taking place. It is a world beyond me. How similar this feels to the early stages of painting.

We return from a long walk in the woods, rain gathering from a light drizzle into thin sheets. You curl up for a nap with the cats and I decide now is a good time to unfold the paintings. They are scattered across the garden, in small piles under the concrete slabs. The unkempt grass has grown up and around the sides, so when I lift them there are a series of near-grassless patches dotted across the lawn like the last squares of a supersize chessboard in a derelict site taken back over by nature. You will not like this.

The folded paintings are almost too heavy to lift, saturated with the water that has also gathered inside. I tip them up and let the excess water empty out. I unfold them one by one. Some have become tough with dried paint, others unravel easily. I lay them out across the garden, creating a huge carpet covering the entire lawn and patio. They are varied in their range of colours and in the ways in which the folds and paint have worked to create surface, texture and marks. At various points are marks reminiscent of Rorschach tests, roughly symmetrical inkblots, or the kind of butterfly pattern a child might make in primary school. One resembles a flattened-out stag's skull, bone-white over dark, dusky purple, another a huge stingray. The paint blooms, the stingray with a solid centre and amorphous edges. Its form clings temporarily to this state and place. It glides off, arrested in the process of transmutation, moving from one thing to another.

Where the folds have been pressed flat by weight and pressure, the lines are more defined. They tend to cut diagonally across swathes of the huge canvases. They create a series of defined borders, diagonals which divide and create space, both across the picture plane and through it, a matrix of optical depths. The softness of the edges, the way that paint often fans out in a rough symmetry either side, gives the sense of a threshold which has been crossed. There is no clear logic to the compositions, and the flattened canvas creates an estrangement, the marks speaking uncannily to the manner in which they were made. These divides create an architecture for the underworld, both picturing it and constructing it. It takes me back to Ovid's opening of *Metamorphoses*:

In nova fert animus mutatas dicere formas/corpora

I'm intrigued by the different translations of this opening line, which I run through Google Translate:

*In the novel, the mind brings about changing forms/
bodies*

The word 'novel' could be replaced with the word 'painting', or the underworld. In the painting, in the underworld, the mind brings about changing forms/bodies.

Certainly the paintings have formed themselves. One surface printing on to another. Paint pulled from one layer to the next, pushed from one surface to another. The paint does not just sit on the surface but has soaked through the unprimed canvases. In these passages of paint, forms shift suddenly from solidity to a gas-like state, as if the paint was able, in its slow spread and drying, to refute its existence as a liquid. In other places its prior liquidity could not be clearer, like the splitting earth on the riverbed of a dried-out tributary. Elsewhere, where the paint retains some gloss, it is seemingly still in the process of spreading through the fabric. Fluidity overcomes fixity. At various points the paintings seem like portals to a submerged world: views into water, reflections on the surface of water, and views from inside the swell of an ocean.

To see this array of bodies and spaces unfolding from the canvases is to feel that life is hatching in the dark. It dedicates a trust to the process. What of you, where do you lie in these folds? I think of you always, at each stage of the making. I am exploring the paintings, led by desire, led by the pull of the other, the pull of you, the desire to see you. I am working towards the place that you are, a place which might be beyond reach, might not yet have opened itself up. The final destination is you, even if it remains an unreachable point. I am never alone in the process of making, however solitary the engagement with the canvas. The voice of an absent figure calls me forwards, deeper.

I have been in the garden for a few hours, as soaked through as the canvases. The rain is steaming off my skin through my sodden shirt. It is only when I go inside that I start to shiver. I take myself upstairs to climb into bed with you, to feel your warm skin against mine, to nest in together as you gently come back from a nap that had turned into a long sleep. Arm around you, I rest my hand on your belly, feel the softness of your skin give, the gentle rise and fall of your breath.

Earlier, walking in the woods, I had noticed your attentiveness. You'd regularly stop, noticing something, bend down to try and identify it, some plant or some kind of fungus. The world seems to suddenly get closer to you, amplified, more alive. The fungi that emerge from the forest floor are mere fragments, the fruit of entire mycological systems underneath the surface, spaces of remarkable complexity and growth beneath our feet. Different forms of patterning consciousness, beyond the human, which weave a web of connectivity together beneath the soil. Eurydice fell to her death in the middle of a forest. She sank into the underworld through the forest floor's mycological mazes.

The artist Aimée Parrott tells me that while pregnant a lot of the pieces she was working on referenced growth and doubles, even before she knew she was having twins. The majority of her works are quite small, normally paintings on calico that combine staining, monoprinting and stitching. The iconography she incorporates into her work varies and is often consciously slippery, ranging from images of the body in the bath, leaves, seed pods, abstract stormy swirls to the inside of the body, mouths and caves. Elsewhere souls are sheets of rain, the suggestion of a moon that becomes a cell, or a body which becomes a volcano, horizon lines become stitched scars or a mycological tendril roots out to read as a vein of blood or a tributary of a river. We can be spun between spatial registers within seconds. One image she posts on Instagram stands out, its iconography more explicit, at least initially. A pair of wings fill the picture plane, hovering above stains of red and purple paint. It is titled, simply, *Mother*.

Parrott and I were represented by the same gallery, and have some close mutual friends. But our contact has been entirely online, mostly through Instagram: digital acquaintances. My engagement with her work was mediated though the small screen of my phone. For all the talk of how the digital landscape can cause alienation, it can also create points of connection and, perhaps more troubling, a blurring of the lines between public and private.

I remember when you posted an image with a caption about our loss to Instagram. I found a deep comfort in the shared kindness of family, friends and even strangers, in this virtual community. But I also felt as if the outside world had flooded into our home, our lives and our grief. Navigating the digital space can be disorientating, creating unexpected transgressions. When I first encountered Parrott's *Mother* painting I found myself wanting to get inside it. I asked Parrott for more information, and for links to any relevant texts on her work or materials. She sent some. But my hunger and desire for connection reached further; I wanted to know about the biographical circumstances around the work and had to catch myself, realising the dangers inherent in this desire.

It was naïve to presume that biographical information would be some kind of key. But more troublingly, of course I had no right to ask for this information. The painting might be public, but it was also deeply personal and private. The connection between biography and painting is not simply joining the dots. Instead, I returned to the painting as primary source.

It's an image rich in ambivalence, containing a female space and experience; one that consciously keeps certain things beyond reach. It's small, 35x45cm, a monotype on calico, introducing a mixture of embroidery and ink and mounted in a sapele tray frame. Wings fill the majority of the frame, drawn with three distinct types of mark. Two reddish-brown smears form a V shape, both coming from the top edge of the canvas to about two-thirds of the way down, meeting in the middle, the shape sitting just to the centre-left of the picture plane. The bottom is curved, reddish-pink, shaped like a valley. Then a series of sinuous triangles fan out to the left and right edges of the frame, creating the impression of wings and feathers, drawn in a series of red dashes, made by sewing a red thread of cotton through the back of the calico, leaving small gaps between the end of each line to create a startling staccato effect. The centre reveals the surface beneath. The wings seem to hover above this space. We read the form and conceptualise a solidity to the wings, while they remain transparent. There is both weight and lightness to them: simultaneously corporeal and ethereal.

Behind this outline are washes of ink and monoprinted surfaces. At the top edge of the painting is a dark-purple strip which reaches across the entire width of the canvas, but rather than soaking across the edge it is held tantalisingly short, the purple ink tracing a frilled, uneven line along this edge. As the purple ink spreads down the calico, it forms a band which fades out across a stitched undulating line. Beneath is a faint upward jolt of umber, seeming to fade into the material, at points only just present. At the bottom of the picture plane is a mound-like shape, the colour of drying blood. The space between these zones at the top and bottom initially appears fairly empty, almost entirely stripped back to the bare cream of the calico. Yet the more we look, the more marks and colours are floating there. In the centre there is a barely visible orb of blue, the pigment clinging to the weave of the fabric, like a shimmering, reflected glimpse of sky. To the right of this nebulous shape is a slightly denser collection of ink, shifting from blue to yellow to magenta, the first or final glimmers of a rainbow, but slightly muddier, filtered through earth. When looking really closely, you see a number of thin, ghostly lines, like delicate threads of blue, red and brown, barely there at all.

Parrott often splits her work into zones with a horizontal division halfway up the canvas. In *As Above, So Below* there is a shell-like outline across the divide, filling the majority of the frame. In the top half, through the shell we see the shape of a female body, two breasts and the curved, rising mound of a pregnant belly. Two triangles of dragged grey paint sit underneath this, suggestive of both open legs and architecture. Beneath the dividing line the marks, colours and forms are of a different register, almost breaking entirely into abstraction. The green, red and grey expressive lines of paint swirl, shape and circumnavigate forms that I struggle to give certain identity to.

In *The Bath* the split between zones is even more stark. In the top half two white arches protrude out of a blue-grey, legs rising out of bathwater from the top of the leg to the curve of the knee, seen as if from the perspective of the bather. In the background, a wall of red and a dark circle that reads as the plughole, but is loose enough to carry other readings. Beneath the halfway line a paler pink suffuses the fabric, two circular forms float over each other: shell-like spirals, or petals flowing and spinning from within, as if contained by some centrifugal force. An ether surrounds these forms, dashed curves of red and orange, thick, bending lines of semi-transparent purple, diffusing at the edges, spinning and swimming their way to the picture's edge. One of the discs breaches the divide between the two spaces, emerging from the bottom, interlacing with the grey of the bathwater, as if just breaking the surface. This small detail provides the dramatic key to the painting. The top half shows the body in the world, in the domestic space of the bath. Beneath the line we are in a far less certain space and place. Is this a microscopic expressive rendering of the internal landscape of the pregnant body? The shell-like forms read as eggs, seeds, spinning discs, the womb. Whatever the space, it is one below, one inside, one not fully known, not absolutely certain.

Both these paintings, and their views of the female body, remind me of Titian's *Poesie*. Titian and his studio made versions of the *Danaë* composition (*c.*1544–1560s). In each, Danaë reclines naked on a bed, legs spread, Jupiter arriving through the window as a shower of golden coins. In one version her hand clearly parts her sex in permission, lets the transformed god enter her and impregnate her. Titian's painting at least gives Danaë centre stage, breathing more life into her than Ovid. In *Metamorphoses* her story is a side note, a useful bit of context in the heroic quest of her son, Perseus. In the midst of high drama, as Perseus is attempting to save Andromeda from the hungry mouth of a sea monster and the waves, he divulges his backstory, presenting himself as slayer, saviour and suitor. A fragment of a sentence is used to present Danaë's story, as an illustration to explain how Perseus came to have wings and to exist in a state between god and mortal:

... son of Jupiter and that Danaë, imprisoned in the
brazen tower, whom Jupiter filled
with his rich golden shower ...

Danaë's father, King Acrisius, had attempted to avoid the prophecy of an oracle. He was told he would never have a male heir but that his daughter, Danaë, would, and that he would be killed by his grandson. King Acrisius had his architects construct a tall bronze chamber, with no doors or windows to enter or exit, and imprisoned Danaë within the chamber. Yet Jupiter, arch shape-shifter, desired her, and so transformed himself into a shower of golden coins, allowing him to enter the building and to enter her. The few words Perseus uses in Ovid's account are telling. *His rich golden shower* is both a literal description of the god's state, but is also loaded with bodily and sexual potency, the god a glittering, golden ejaculatory form.

In Titian's painting the hand which parts and the nature of the pose allow for a moral ambiguity, a complicity on the part of Danaë. The convenient compliance of the female victim a device to circumnavigate the horror of rape. Danaë's eyes look longingly upwards, her body reclines with a relaxed abandon, she is openly partaking in the action and in one version a small dog is curled up asleep beside her. Dogs play a major role in the drama of Titian's paintings, and here its calm reverie suggests that the arrival of this visitor, both Jupiter as the shower of coins or the viewer, is not seen as a threat.

In his iconic text *The Lives of the Artists* Titian's contemporary Giorgio Vasari wrote what many cite as the first art history textbook, a biography of the lives and works of major artists of the Italian Renaissance. It is split chronologically into three sections to construct a narrative of progression ending with the High Renaissance and the genius of Michelangelo. It argues an inevitability of evolution, with other artists situated as pawns to Michelangelo's king. Vasari recounts the story of visiting Titian's studio with Michelangelo and seeing one of the Danaë paintings. They praise the work in front of Titian, but on leaving their praise is coloured by a particular bias. Vasari recounts Michelangelo's observation,

> *saying that his colouring and his manner much pleased him, but that it was a pity that in Venice men did not learn to draw well from the beginning, and that those painters did not pursue a better method in their studies.*

It's a loaded statement that carries within it a neat synopsis of the divide of ideologies between Titian and Michelangelo, and more broadly between Venice and Central Italy, between *colorito* and *desegno*. For Vasari and Michelangelo, drawing was the foundation of painting, and art in general. To draw was to design, to lay the aesthetic, intellectual and compositional framework of a work of art. There was also a gendering in the split, and Titian's tendency towards the paintings of the reclining female nude as opposed to the erect, active male fitted this crude binary. They were arguing that in the choice of subject matter, in the lack of polish in his under drawing and therefore presumably by default the openness and fluidity of his painterly process, he was making something fundamentally inferior. The inferiority was, without doubt, given a gendered dimension. Titian, and the wider Venetian style, was considered more feminine. It is strange to frame the paintings and this split in such simplistic gender binaries, particularly as the power balance lies still with the male gaze.

Parrott's compositions spin the perspective, positioning the lens from the viewpoint of the pictured figure, making our view hers. Parrot unites us; makes painter, subject and viewers inhabit the same space, the same body. These paintings are female at an experiential level. We are submerged and enveloped by it. The paintings act on us, not us on them.

I wonder whether my entering that space, in my view of the work or in these words, is to reassert the same penetrative gaze and desire that Titian's *Danaë* presents. Perhaps the male gaze can't penetrate Parrott's works. Perhaps we are seeing into them, while also remaining outside them.

A number of her marks in *Mother* are monoprinted. Parrot paints directly on to a copper plate, drawing on the V-shaped lines that form the split of the wings and the red dashes that make up the mound at the base of the fabric. The ink is unfixed, which provides malleability at every stage of the process, allowing the marks to be added, removed and reworked until she is happy with the flow of the lines, the colour and the placement. Sarah Kate Wilson remarks that this *sustained period of malleability appeals to her*. Even though Parrot is utilising a printing process, her approach is distinctly painterly. That is, she embraces the process as open, the destination unfixed.

The unstretched calico is carefully placed over the copper plate and then run through a press, where the pressure presses the ink not just on to but into the unprimed fabric. The presence of pigment in the weave shifts not only the materiality of the final painting but how we view it, how the object and image function. In the final painting we see how the marks, and therefore the form of the wings and the mound, appear to be at a slight distance. It is not a distance created only by illusion, but a literal one. The paint is just beyond us, embedded into the weave. The marks and forms hover in soft focus, a hazed space.

This technique recalls a scene in *Throne of Blood*, the 1957 film by Japanese filmmaker Akira Kurosawa. His reimagining of Shakespeare's *Macbeth* is filmed in black and white, suffused with fog. In a world stripped of colour, the fog's obfuscation of space is all-encompassing. It becomes a character. The fog is the space of the supernatural, danger, the traumatic erosion of memory, the threat of unseeable futures. The film is centred around dramatic and existential discombobulation and what it means to be lost. At one point the camera is fixed, as two equestrian figures navigate a thick fog. The horses trot into and out of, to and from total obscurity. The way the horses vanish and then reappear and the soft dissolution of presence reminds me of Parrott's work, particularly *Mother*.

When the copper plate and calico are removed from the press, the majority of the ink has been transferred from plate to fabric, but not all of it. Some remains on the plate, and this provides Parrot with a site of retrieval, an opportunity for reworking and remixing. An exact repeat of the previous print isn't the outcome, rather a further stage in the process of evolution. Parrott calls the reused plate a ghost print, the ghost of the old print informing the next one. As Wilson states, *familial echoes bind her works together*, repeating marks and motifs, reappearing across a body of work in new guises, with new intensities, as if she is creating her own painterly genealogy. When the same plate is reused on the same canvas she is interested in the stutter in the transformations that take place. Often the slip of the fabric or the plate will create a repositioning of the marks; a misalignment, or realignment. Faint traced marks create an echo, a temporal complexity, like a double exposure in photography.

The most striking aspect of the painting is the red thread. The stitches draw our attention to its materiality, to the fragility of its surface, now punctuated by this array of tiny holes. They become the focus of the composition. Perhaps this explains the myopia of my vision. I had only seen the wings, had missed the explicit presence of a female body at the bottom of the painting. Once seen, the axis of the painting spins, and spins us with it. We are transcendently above ground, beyond flesh and into the space of spirit, while also being below ground, beneath water, encased in the solidity of corporeality. One form emerges from another, two lives inextricably linked and made from the same matter. It codifies the nature of motherhood, specifically motherhood during pregnancy. Those wings, suggestive of angels, point not so much towards the model of *Danaë* but the model of the Annunciation. The angel, rather than the messenger of divine intervention, is the miraculous life force of the mother and of the baby.

Parrott's paintings gather meaning when we read them in a series of multiple canvases within one body of work. Marks, iconography and ideas reappear and shift. Jack Smurthwaite uses the word *convergent* to describe this instability of iconography in Parrott's work, suggesting a conscious malleability. In Ovid's *Metamorphoses* humans and gods are constantly threatened by or threatening with transformation, and Parrott's poetics place us in even more unstable territory, never letting anything settle into an angular form. Shapes form and dissipate, exist and become inexistent.

To exist in one moment and then to not. Eurydice inhabits a perpetual cycle of this state. In retelling after retelling, her tragic plight is coded into the structure of the myth. Imagine Eurydice not as pen-on-paper as fictional construct but as flesh and bone, a human full of breath and agency. Each time her story is retold is a reincarnation, a set of parallel universes built by writer after writer. Each time she's sent to death, each time she is offered the hope of return, each time it is stolen from her right at the threshold.

This is the fragile point we found ourselves in during those first few days after each positive test. The earliest stages of pregnancy are unstable, and a form that would become human but was in these cellular states of splitting, hatching and implanting, was in the process of crossing into being. In these early days our minds were hatching possibility. I feared the opposite movement. I see you longing, hoping that things are continuing to grow inside you, that the hatch might be opening further.

The word *hatch* links our hopes and your body to ideas of the home, and signals to me the lazy slide to deficient language that is often used around pregnancy, both medically and colloquially. The body as a home, the body as a host; implying a separation which doesn't acknowledge the deep and complex network between the body of the mother and the matter which is from her body, of her body and in relation to her body. I don't think of your body as a home. It is something more intimate and entangled.

In the days after the positive test I notice you suspended, held in a state of waiting. You appear partially frozen, caught in a cycle of testing a couple of times a day, to seek a physical, visible reassurance for the invisible happening inside you. Today is no different. The white sheets of the mattress still hold your warmth. I barely notice it at first, just a small smudge on the sheets, but then the redness of it catches my attention. It is unmistakably a blood stain, no bigger than a fifty-pence piece. At almost the same time I hear you call my name, quietly. I come straight to you and you keep repeating my name, stuck on it, can't get beyond the plea. Then, *I'm bleeding*, holding up a tissue with another small smear of blood. You won't let go of the tissue. I kneel down on the floor in front of the loo and hold you. We say nothing, my head in your lap, your head on mine, wrapped into each other.

In the coming days what we already knew is confirmed. The

tests get weaker, chemical traces of a line confirming a pregnancy that no longer exists. You keep testing. I can feel you
slipping inside yourself, away from the world, away from me.
By the time your period comes you are almost relieved. *Better it
was early*, people keep telling us, keep translating the pregnancy
into abstracted medical language. *A chemical pregnancy*, they say.
It was barely a thing, just a cluster of cells, a ball of matter. As if
we are all not just clusters of cells, balls of matter.

5

Eurydice

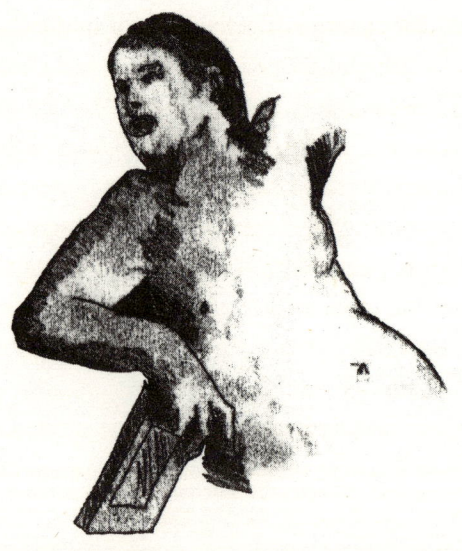

We start trying again as soon as we can and you become pregnant again. But the pattern repeats, and within days there is bleeding, a loss. It's strange how quickly the grief we felt before shifts to resignation. It's almost like we expected it, and any feelings that are there seem softer, or perhaps just buried. Before, even if I felt you growing distant, I could sense the scale of your feelings. Now you seem closed off not just to me, but to any emotions. We have grown barriers. We have come to assume the worst.

We're referred to the recurrent miscarriage clinic and put

under the care of an expert. A number of tests are done but no abnormalities are found, so the suggestion is we *just keep trying*. In these moments we become aware of the limitations of modern science. Western medicine is astonishing at diagnosing and treating a medical problem that can be identified. Yet when there is a problem that can't be named, it falls back on the bluntest of language. We give ourselves over again to blind faith, but are convinced that there is an issue that can't be located.

The next month you are pregnant again. It is clear the issue is not about getting pregnant, but staying so. The red line leaves us feeling ambivalent, full of fear as much as hope, almost complacent in our certainty that it is a holding pattern ahead of another loss. Yet in the coming days the line gets stronger, and there is no sign of blood. It appears, for now, that it is sticking. You picture it as a tree spreading roots inside yourself, and at night I speak into your belly, hope that words act like water, feeding these roots.

And then, pain. We are booked in for a scan at the Early Pregnancy Unit, and the wait seems to stretch out in front of us, everything on pause in the meantime. I see your words dry up, notice your energy shift into a state close to slumber as you google obsessively, take painkillers safe for pregnancy. You're on autopilot, a knotted ball. Covid laws have shifted and I can come to the scan. In the waiting room you squeeze my hand tightly. Through the window there is a view on to the playground, where a mother holds her baby's hands as it takes clumsy steps, like a concentrated drunk, a toppling imitation of walking. The framing of the view feels like a picture of a future we might not be able to have.

We are called through to the scanning room. They pull the blue curtain for you to get ready. I fold your underwear, and you laugh at this pointless gesture, wince as the pain in your stomach pulls. You lie back, open yourself, we breathe together.

Your hand and face tighten in discomfort as they look. Nothing. Another nurse tries, and the silence is occasionally punctuated by her talking us through what she is looking for. She tells us this is quite common, that there might be nothing to worry about, that at such an early stage it is often hard or even close to impossible to get an image of the foetus. *This is*, she says, *what we call a pregnancy of unknown location.* They calmly explain the next steps, that they will test your HCG levels and book us in for another scan in a week, when they will retest them. We hold on to this, to the possibility of those levels rising, to the fact that by the next scan there will be something to see. *They are probably just hiding from us*, the sonographer says. *Try to not lose hope, this is not uncommon.*

In the gap between scans the pain persists but there is a drip feed of change which unknots you. You've begun to feel sick, can explain the pains as the expansion of your uterus, *though maybe I'm becoming a wimp*, you frown. *It really hurts.* A week later, the repeat test confirms your HCG levels have been rising at the rate they would expect in the early stages of a pregnancy. We cry, relief like a drink of fresh water. *It's okay*, I whisper, as much to myself. *It's going to be okay.* We return to the scan filled with hope. We know that by now something will be visible. A yolk sac, perhaps a heartbeat.

The waiting room, the walk to the scan, the curtain, are all familiar by now. You breathe yourself calm as they insert the probe. I feel you tense up and go a little light-headed myself, powerless next to your vulnerability, how open you have to be to these intimate invasions.

The scan seems to go on forever. At first the two nurses fall silent, and then another is called. There is lots of coded talk, lots of knowing sounds and signals as they look at the screen. I place my forehead against yours. You are clammy, crying quietly. *It's okay, it's okay. I love you, I love you. Breathe deeply, focus on your breath.* The nurses inform us that they are unable to see the foetus, so it is still a pregnancy of unknown location, but that at this stage this is not what they would expect. They check the record of your HCG levels to confirm the consistent rise. There is a chance, or even a likelihood, they say, that this is an ectopic pregnancy. Buzzing rises in my ears. This was a possibility you raised early in this pregnancy, when the pain in your stomach got sharper. But I promised you it wouldn't be. Couldn't be. You'd already been through so much, it could not happen to you, to us. But the nurse is talking urgently, calmly, explaining that the blastocyst may have implanted itself in the right fallopian tube. If it is this, it cannot be rescued and cannot survive. We are quietly moved into another room, given Covid tests in case of a hospital visit and told to wait while they consult over next steps.

It all happens very slowly, and then very quickly. We are stuck alone in the new room for an hour. You won't speak. Occasionally someone pops back in, to pick up our tests, to offer a glass of water, to let us know they are still trying to work out what they've seen, and they are waiting on a call back from the clinician. We don't have a sense of what is going on. I make the mistake of googling ectopic pregnancy, and see that if left untreated it can rupture and cause a life-threatening haemorrhage to the mother. I try to keep you distracted, to stop you from making a similar search. Your pain gets stronger, your face paler, and the word *haemorrhage* reverberates in my head.

A nurse enters with a performed calmness, but there seems to be the edge of a panic. They tell us you need go to hospital, and that the clinician thinks you will need to undergo surgery immediately. *We could call an ambulance, but if you have a car I wouldn't wait.* The journey is a blur, and you seem almost catatonic. I talk and talk, can't shut up, desperate to penetrate your thickening shell. The fear is calcifying around you. In my worry about you, I have no thought to spare for what is about to happen – another loss, another possibility taken. When we arrive there is nowhere to park, and I pull up on a grassy verge under a sycamore, helicopter seeds spinning on to the windshield. I want to stop time, to hold you, but this is an emergency. You are deep inside yourself now – I have to undo your seatbelt, pull your coat around your shoulders. You say something as I urge you towards the women's centre entrance. *What?* You repeat yourself: *it's my birthday in two days. I need to cancel the party.*

I'm trying to guide us to the right department but keep getting us lost in the hallways of the hospital. I hate myself in that moment, my ineptitude, my impotence. I keep telling you *it's fine, it's fine. It's just around the corner,* but you can't hear me, and I am outside my body, I am a camera looking down on to this scene of two figures wandering aimlessly around the corridor in some dark romcom in which a man loses his wife to a haemorrhage in a hospital hallway because he has no basic sense of direction. Like a murderous version of the clichéd bumbling Brit. *I'm awfully sorry, my ineptitude appears to have killed you.*

We eventually find the right department, press the button to be let in. There is no one at the desk so we press another button and sit in the waiting room. We wait again, in total silence. A nurse comes out and takes you through the locked door. Covid rules mean I am not allowed with you. Apparently I shouldn't even be in the waiting room. So you are led away and I am sent outside, in the dark over what is going to happen and when. As you go through the double doors into the ward you look back. I mouth *I love you.*

I find my way back to the car park. We stay in touch via text and over the coming minutes it becomes clear what is going to happen. They have done a series of checks and confirmed an ectopic pregnancy. They are going to take you into surgery immediately to remove one of your tubes. You are so scared, but we're unable to talk on the phone. I'm half grateful for the tonelessness of text, so you won't hear my own fear. You warn me they are about to get you ready for surgery, so we will fall out of communication. *It will be a few hours. I'll text you when I'm back.*

I need to tell your parents, my own. I don't know how to start, so break it down to the barest essentials, bullet points almost. As I type, the words start to sink in. As soon as they're sent, the questions come back. I reply as fast as I can, turn my phone on to silent and sit back for a few moments. Heat rises from my belly to my brain and I scream into the steering wheel, cry until my head aches and my eyes sting. I have never felt so far away from safety.

This is what I do while I wait. I drive home, back to the studio, to the unfolded, unstretched canvases. Relics from the time before: before our cells lodged in your tube, before those scans, the false hope, before you looked back and I couldn't follow. They are hung around the studio, pinned to walls, tacked from the ceiling, wrapped over supporting beams. In a few instances I have used burnt stretcher bars recovered from the fire as poles to drape them from. I stand among them and breathe in paint and turps. I check my phone – barely any time has passed. Messages are stacking up from family, close friends, but I only want to hear from you. *It will be a few hours.* I set my alarm for an hour's time. One hour, to step back to before.

Like the burnt paintings, what interests me about these unstretched canvases is the removal of a frame, the lifting of them from the flatness of a wall. Suddenly the form I had used as a default seemed so limiting. The rectangular frame of stretched canvas felt closed off, a bordered world, one contained and controlled. The frame acting not just to regulate the space but to create a window on to another world, a realm beyond us. The frame created a division between what is inside the painting and our place outside it. Made the threshold between those spaces solid and certain.

I liked the sudden opening up of the space by the canvas not being stretched tight, how it turned these canvases into more slippery things, part sculpture and part painting. But more than this, they started to take on other readings, as if their form and function were not explicitly clear. And the slightest shift in how they were hung changed this. To lift them off the wall and into the space of the studio shifted the mode of engagement. As the canvases had been unprimed the relationship between their front and back is one of direct consequence, the marks of both seeping into each other, like the recto and verso of a page in a book. However thick the paint, these consequences were still at play, as the acrid and destructive quality of the materials I had added meant that paint which had seeped through one side would eat away at the paint on the other side, a body devouring itself from within, forms falling and rising up through the surface and picture plane.

Hung across the studio, the paintings look like loose sheets from a huge, unbound book. The doubling cancels any notion of front and back, and by their nature they can never be fully encountered or occupied by the gaze. We can only access half the painting, we cannot possess it completely. To see one side is to not be able to see the other. In Jean Cocteau's film *Orphée* (1950) the underworld is accessed through a mirror. Orpheus eventually finds his way through the solid space of the mirror, where glass seems to shift into liquid state, where his reflection becomes the image to enter. These paintings feel like something similar, entrances and exits, the viewer only able to occupy one space. Eurydice, the absent other, is the unseen figure standing on the other side of the fabric, obscured from view. The two figures, present and absent, look into the opposite sides of the canvas. We are at that edge, but we cannot reach in.

You, looking back as the double doors close. *I'll text you when I'm back.* In these hours the distance from you feels impossibly cavernous, unbreachable. Perhaps Eurydice, perhaps you, can be found among my swaying canvases and their double faces. Perhaps there is an underworld to explore there, in every fold, in the looking back, in the falls beneath the divides, beyond me.

The waiting is insufferable, and time drags slowly. I can't escape that image of you, the doors closing, the look, the disappearance. Going through, to go under. Still no news, so I break from the paintings to do some reading. There is a stack of research books in the studio, in my office, dotted around the house. In the sitting room there is a little pile of books and printed articles on the artist Bracha Ettinger. I've not shown you her work yet, and I feel a slight trepidation. Perhaps it will be too raw, entering as it does the space you have had to occupy during the pregnancies. I find myself diving into images of paintings, as if somehow searching for you there, in the depths of these imagined underworlds.

Bracha Ettinger is a shape-shifter, what could be lazily labelled as a polymath. There is a gravitational pull to her creative output. I was drawn in by a large series of paintings she made titled *Eurydice*. I reached out to her through email, with no expectation to hear back. But a few days later I did, and upon reflection recognise there is a quiet radicalism to this. Her critical thinking, psychoanalytical investigations and her art practice are exercises in connectivity and empathy. This warmth is not a form of frictionless acquiescence, but fights against the forms of separation and hierarchy that the institutional apparatus of her various roles – artist, activist, psychoanalytical practitioner, Jew, mother – perpetuate. Her generosity and openness are political, ethical, creative and critical acts.

Yet her paintings are veiled, always beyond us. Paradoxes lie at the heart of everything she does. Among the material she sent me is a PDF of a cross-disciplinary magazine, *Nova Express*, which has just released a special edition on her practice. The magazine includes a series of photographs taken by the artist Maria Luigia Gioffre of Ettinger in her studio. In one we see Ettinger posing on a ladder, in the distance the steps which lead down into the basement space. The symbolism of the ladder and the steps is not lost, speaking as they do to the descent and rise of Eurydice, to the studio space as a metonym for the underworld, and vice versa. Everything is carefully staged, and it is even noted in the caption to the photograph that the paintings 'on display' in the image are shrouded. Here is a game of simultaneously revealing and conceding, of opening up a private space to the public gaze, but not fully. It is a practice Ettinger has followed with the *Eurydice* works. Produced as they are in serialisation over many years, she tends to veil the incomplete works when visitors come. The veiling is revealing. They are not removed from site, nor covered with a completely opaque material, but rather a semi-transparent layer, providing a tantalising glimpse of the surfaces beneath. Theatricality veers towards religiosity, veils shrouding sacred, secret spaces beyond witness.

The magazine includes reproductions of a number of the complete *Eurydice* paintings, but an accidental veiling has also occurred here. I have downloaded the PDF and printed it out on our black and white printer. The printing is clumsy, the mechanistic lines of ink pulled across the surface still clearly visible, articulating the ways in which the image is brought into being. The ink sits heavily on the page, the tone pushed up a notch. It is as if the images have dropped back into darkness, or been smeared over by the printer's functionality. Like the veils in the studio they are shrouded, but here by inky darkness on paper, as opposed to translucent white veils of fabric.

What should we make of this veiling, both the deliberate and accidental? The veiling of sight, of desire. Veils are suggestive of curtains, or netting around a bed, or clothes and lingerie. The home, the bed, the body obscured, interplays of transparency and opacity to lure the eye in, to keep it out. The reduction to shape, space left for the imagination, a play between what is seen and what is beyond sight. Desire is the eye's keenness for touch.

In 1558, right in the midst of the time he was working on the *Poesie* paintings, Titian produced one of the strangest canvases of his career. The *Portrait of Cardinal Filippo Archinto* is striking, depicting the cardinal robed, sitting in a chair, but with the majority of his face and half his body obscured by a semi-transparent curtain. It gathers in tight folds at the fringes, meaning his facial features are particularly obscured. Archinto was a diplomat, papal bureaucrat, bishop and lawyer. He had the trust and support of Emperor Charles V and Pope Paul III, and later Philip II, which led to a frictionless ascent through the corridors of power, moving fluidly upwards into positions of increasing prestige. At the end of 1556 he was appointed as the Archbishop of Milan by Pope Paul IV, but was unable to take up the post due to the Spanish governor not believing that the move was supported by Philip II. The distrust between the political powers led to long delays, and he would die in June 1558, shortly before he was due to finally take up the post. What to make of the portrait, painted in the midst of this uncertainty, unclear if it comes just before or just after his death?

Renaissance portraiture was founded on a belief that painting was able to reach beyond the seen, beyond mere representation of appearances. The painter could translate the sitter's inner world, both psychological and spiritual, into paint. They could give the soul solid form. To look at the portrait is to look for clues: in pose, in iconography, in the handling of paint, not just to what this person looked like but who they were.

What does Titian's veiling tell us? A face just visible, one eye almost entirely out of sight, the other almost covered, the uncovered half looking out at us, our gaze returned. Both subject and viewer are behind a ghostly curtain. One hand holds a book, the other sits at the edge of the veil, drawing our eye to the ring on his finger. He is placed between power and obscurity, between certainty and the unknown. Is this the place of his political limbo or the place between life and death? Which of these places are we both looking from and into? It is this that Titian and Ettinger are interested in portraying. Places of ambiguity and ambivalence, thresholds between states, where the relationship between subject and viewer, artist and canvas, is made consciously mysterious.

It is in the movement from life and into death that Ettinger's *Eurydice* paintings reside. Let's return first to Eurydice, to a figure sent to death, into the inescapable underworld. The power of grief, desire and her voice: agents that pull Orpheus into that space. Their joint ascent, the reversal of who is following whom, rising towards the light, the surface, life. Yet in looking back Orpheus returns her to death. What is in this look and action? What of Eurydice, what she sees and experiences?

Ettinger begins with materials that already carry weight. These might be pages of scanned text in Hebrew and French, snippets sourced from books, art-historical imagery, photographs from a personal family collection and from historical archives. Images of family gatherings in the Lodz Ghetto before the Holocaust, or images of Ukrainian women and children being sent to execution. Photographs made intense by the knowledge of what sits outside that moment, in the future. Photographs as physical things don't just collect history, they collect meaning through personal association, through what follows, through the history that unfolds after that moment. A seemingly mundane image of family life in the Lodz Ghetto becomes loaded with the horror of what's to come.

Ettinger starts by partially photocopying the source material. She lays the image on to the screen of the machine, lets the light of the scanner pull across it, waits for the printer to start converting information into ink. Then she pauses the process. She opens up the printer in the midst of printing, catching the image as the ink is being pulled across the page, still wet, the toner tacky on the paper's surface. The ink, and therefore the image, are yet to be bound to the paper by heat. The image is neither complete nor fixed.

Arresting this journey of the original to copy is interesting. In the space between two replicas is an image facing in two directions. It is a suspension, and an opening up, of time. The image has not become what it should have become. The image pulled from the printer is a refracted, blurred trace, not of a lost past but a lost future. It appears to shimmer. There is a trembling sense of an overwriting having taken place, when the opposite is true. The image gives the impression of erasure, yet something is still to be laid down.

With the ink still wet the image becomes smudged in the process of removal and then deliberately. Paint drags, suggests a blur. The blur exists in photography, the indicator of a form moving through time as the shutter closes, capturing the ghostly trails of motion. But the blur cannot exist in painting in the same way. The photographic source run through the photocopier exists in a halfway house between photograph and painting, the blur functioning in the painterly sense of recording the shift of matter while recalling the blur in a photo. Here figures are being moved in ways they were not moving, being moved both into and out of existence. The blur gives the appearance of disappearing and degeneration, but it is also appearing.

Ettinger then paints over these surfaces, predominantly using single-haired brushes, to allow the most delicate of lines of paint. She builds up paint in straight lines, vertical and then horizontal, one colour at a time, her hand replicating the machine. Paint is applied and then rubbed off in semi-transparent layers of oil paint. Sometimes she adds toner from the cartridge to the paint. Stage by stage the image disappears and then reappears, in a process of loss and recovery.

Everything is done with care. The brush is a needle, the paint its thread, line after line. Griselda Pollock labels Ettinger a *curator of wounds*, but she is also a healer of wounds, the brush both scarring the surface and stitching it. Touch and non-touch play against each other, the hand and the machine conflating each other. As Brian Massumi observes, *it takes time to stop time.* Working on the paintings for years means that time is layered into the surface. The images, in being worked both towards and away from the original source, are floating, *frozen in the unoccupiable in-between of its own becoming.* The word 'frozen' is repeated in the literature about these works. It refers both to stasis and also the way ice holds things in states of flux. The painting is a cryogenic chamber. Or the deepest-blue ice on the planet, compressed, holding light, trapping geological histories.

The source imagery of these paintings is not totally lost,

either visually or in the paintings' content. They connect back to the source, to history and substantially to the communal trauma of the Holocaust. Ettinger enacts the visual equivalent of a contronym, her paintings holding two opposing meanings at once. The word 'cleave' comes to mind. Meaning to cut, to split, but also meaning to hold on to, cling to. Then a third that sits between them, to cleave through, referring to the motion of passing through. Ettinger's *Eurydice* paintings are all three at once. The images in the paintings have been cleaved from history, are cleaving to history and are cleaving through history. Memory takes an unusual form in them, not just attached to what happened, to the violence of the future that awaits the women and children led away in Ukraine, or the horror that would fall upon the families in the Lodz Ghetto. This memory suggests alternative futures, the possibility of hope, a history that didn't happen, that needn't have happened as it did. A parallel universe, another possible world, of light in the dark. The underworld becomes everything that is beyond sight; testimonies are robbed by genocidal death. History itself becomes Eurydice.

For her, vision is murderous, a view codified into these paintings. To see is to die. For Eurydice and these paintings, to see is to be cut from life for a second time. There is a central paradox. Eurydice is seen, and in being seen, is alive, is present. Yet the act of seeing, as Judith Butler states, *pushes her back to death*. To look is to lose again. To be seen is to die again. The irresistible, grasping desire to possess is the very thing that causes the irreversible and permanent separation. Ettinger's paintings bring us into a trapped loop repeating itself over and over. What Butler calls an *irresolvable ambiguity*.

The suggestion of internal worlds, where foetal and female forms meet, makes them the clearest manifestation of her critical thinking around her idea of the Matrixial Borderspace. The space in which gestation, birth and death all collide. As she says, *theory does not exhaust painting; painting does not melt into theory.*

The womb is seen as the definitive space of both strangeness and familiarity. A space we have all occupied but which we cannot and do not know, the ultimate uncanny. In her theory, the womb is not a passive receptacle registering traces, it produces them. The encounter is one of mutual transformation. We are both known and unknown to the other. The mother and baby to be are intimate strangers. This is a primal paradox of existence.

Ettinger challenges the certainty that there is a clear divide between the I and a you. The other – be that lover, baby to be, viewer, artist or painter, Eurydice – is not beyond us but is rather *a partner in difference.*

Ettinger's *Eurydice* paintings are embodiments of the Matrixial Borderspace. You cannot possess a painting, like Orpheus could not possess Eurydice with his gaze. You are one player in the scheme of connections, the viewer as both witness and partner in a process of co-emergence. It is a collective, participatory act of generative continuation and growth passed from stranger to stranger, from lover to lover, from trace to trace, from viewer to painting in a cycle of perpetual reciprocity. To make a painting is to make something that exists in the empty space, that resides at the borderlines, beyond the limits of the self.

Space is the veil from which Eurydice is emerging and fading back into, it is the huge chasm of the underworld and death to which she has come and will return. It is the threshold we are at, both looking into and beyond us.

The dynamic of the gaze is centrifugal, a force spinning inwards towards scattered versions of Eurydice, into a fragmented, veiled underworld. It spins us in and spins us out. The painting is not a passive receiver of our gaze, it contains its own.

In the encounter at the borderspace, the multiple encounter, trails are left. Be that between painter and painting, Orpheus and Eurydice, the viewer and the painting. The exchange is between outside and inside, in which the painting is capable of representing the originally unrepresentable desire of the viewer. This desire then moves between us, connects us, it is an intimate exchange. Like on a Möbius strip, *the artist's desire slides along the strip, which, twisting and turning, also catches the desire of the viewer.*

What if these paintings, if all paintings, work in both directions. If the paintings can hold traces not just of the painter's desire but also the viewer's, if they remain open to receive and be engraved with new trails and traces. On return it leaves all participants changed, imprinted on by the other. It is a meeting point between strangers. As Ettinger says, it *inflames the desire of my eye and of an-other's eye to see.*

It suggests the potential for the shareability of trauma. Even trauma that might have led to erasures, through death or lack of testimony. They are paintings which see us participate in the traumatic events of the other. They suggest that, rather than empathy being an impossibility, instead it is impossible for there *not* to be connection, for there *not* to be forms of sharing. They are paintings which suggest the possibility of the other not being a complete stranger. Of us, like Eurydice and Orpheus, reaching across the divide.

There is, at the very least, in her Eurydice paintings, the hope of entering otherwise inaccessible spaces. Such listening and looking requires deep attention, a form of intimacy which is subversive in its attempts. Perhaps we will listen and there is nothing there, but we should at least try to lean into the silence, into belief.

So much about Ettinger's output articulated my aims. Not only was I was trying to understand what you were experiencing, I was trying to express it in my work.

I had her matrix in mind when looking at the double-sided paintings hanging in my studio. Could they exist in the forever present of their materiality, a present looking both backwards and forwards at once? The backward glance clearly related to all the paintings, including the *Orpheus and Eurydice* works, that had been lost in the studio fire. But in the loss of those paintings there was also a partial erasure of the worlds contained in them, of the wider body of material they related to, of the entire underworld they depicted and constructed. The pre-fire *Orpheus and Eurydice* project had existed across multiple media and in multiple formats. The paintings could stand alone or in association with this wider body of work. In the documentary I made with filmmaker Mark Jones, the paintings became part of the fabric of a fictional world of a version of Orpheus as a painter mourns the loss of Eurydice, painting his memories of the underworld. You recorded a narrative voiceover, a poem from the mouth of Eurydice, a voice speaking from the underworld. In the graphic novel we made, where your poems were scattered as fragments, the voice of Eurydice was presented as lost notes scattered in the underworld that Orpheus entered.

In truth the matrix spreads further. It's a web which covers the entirety of my artistic career. The fire took works from across a twelve-year period. Numerous projects I had considered self-contained with clearly defined parameters. But the uniform destruction of the fire reminded me that the boundaries between projects were porous. Like fire, creativity is a kind of monster that devours everything it comes into contact with.

I wanted to dissolve the divide. I wanted to turn the viewer and artist into protagonists. These new double-sided paintings were emptied of explicit figurations. The relationship between different forms in the work and the surfaces was more complicated. In front of these hung paintings I, and later the viewer, could become Orpheus, and Eurydice became the figure lost inside, or emerging from within.

I look at the surfaces and I see, even in your absence, the possibility of Eurydice. If the past version has faded, this new one is to emerge. It's now that I realise, in my search for sources, that it had been there all along. I wanted to return to your poems, to that voice and architecture of Eurydice's experience, but also to the forms of self that had been translated into them. Reading the poems again, it was odd to see how they contained not just the myth but also your past and, uncannily, your present. The present, the very thing I had been distracting myself from.

My phone beeps. You. *I'm awake. Come.*

Uncertain if this is allowed within the current laws, I'm let on to the ward. This crumbling edifice of a building and institution is stuck together by goodwill. You give me a vague, watery-eyed smile, high from the anaesthetic and painkillers. I pull up a chair, and you tell me the operation has been a success, that they removed your fallopian tube – *I'm a one-tube wonder!* – and the pregnancy along with it. If it had grown any larger it could have haemorrhaged and your life would have been at risk. You are speaking as if half asleep, forcefully cheery and with a remembered script. The language and tone are not your own. You are talking about yourself as if you are a stranger, as if this has happened to another body. You shuffle up the bed and your face contorts in pain, so we press the button to ask for more pain relief.

Over the next couple of hours you are visited a few times for various checks, talked through how to manage the recovery in the coming month. I am studiously ignored, a blind eye turned to my presence. Your cheer continues, but you don't let go of my hand. I wonder how and when you will process all this. That morning we had every reason to be hopeful, and now a part of you and the pregnancy is gone. Eventually you are given the all-clear to go home. Getting out of the bed and into your clothes is a slow and painful task. You try to put your tights on and I stop you. *Your stiches. Oh yes*, you say, absently. I feel certain you have forgotten, or have not yet understood what has happened.

The ward is situated within the same building as the maternity wards, so there are newborn babies at every turn. Each step makes you wince, but you refuse a wheelchair. I take you to the car and return to sort out the parking fee. There are two men outside having a smoke and eating fish and chips. I am incapable of operating the machine, and one of them shouts a few pointers. They are both beaming, tell me one of them has just become a father and the other an uncle, and that they are just refuelling. *What about you mate?* I tell them I was in with my wife, we're just leaving. I'm not sure how it gets lost in translation, but they offer me warm congratulations on the little one. When I get back to the car you are asleep, cheek pressed to the cool glass. I do up your seatbelt and drive us home.

6

Under

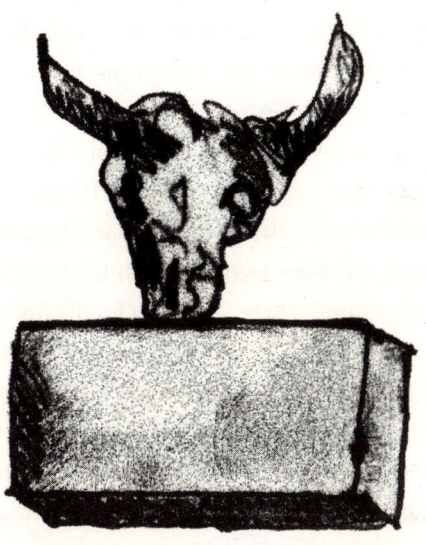

In the weeks of your recovery, as with the twins' miscarriage, we are surprised by the level of your physical pain and discomfort. At first this distracts from attending to what has happened. We are focused on the minutiae of pain relief, moving you from bed to sofa, finding comfortable positions, extra pillows, checking on the surprisingly large and tender wounds left by the surgery. You say you are scared of splitting apart, of the stitches in your belly button reopening. But the real pain waits for you on the other side of your physical recovery, and when it arrives it is on a tide of anger unlike anything I've witnessed from you before.

You are resentful of the pain, the inconvenience, the uselessness of the discomfort and the constant, stinging reminder of what has been lost. This pregnancy, of course, and all the others too – we have to count, to check how many, and this enrages you: that they are this numerous. You fixate on the paperwork you signed before surgery, agreeing to the 'disposal of matter' alongside standard hospital waste. You are mourning your tube, that a part of you is now gone for an awful reason, that it will impact our chances of conception in the future, but we can't quite yet bear to start researching or questioning exactly what the ramifications are. At this stage you are mainly fearful of it happening again, another ectopic in the other tube, and then the opportunity being taken completely from us. You say you have lost the last of your innocence, that now pregnancy feels loaded with danger. You are fearful and distrustful of your own body, it feels like it's failing you. *I feel cursed*, you say. *The rape, the depression, the losses. I'm cursed*. We work at the language, but such attempts feel superficial, decorative rearrangements of how we approach it, the relationship between you and your body has already become terrifyingly toxic.

In the weeks of your physical recovery I watch your mental health decline. The impact of the physical discomfort and limits on your movements make it hard to implement the normal things we would do when I notice you falling. A walk in the woods, a trip to the sea, a swim in the river. Covid has spun another of its lockdowns, meaning we cannot distract you with visits, cannot help stitch these wounds with friends, with your long-planned, year-delayed birthday party. In bed you try to get comfortable, only able to fall asleep when Luna, our cat, curls into the curve of your legs and purrs. You are sleeping more and more in the days, in part from the pain, but in part to absent yourself. It is years since I've seen you like this, and last time the descent took you into a space so dark you overdosed. My fear mounts and mounts.

Reading through your old Eurydice poems, I am struck by how, for all their rooting in myth, they are so firmly embedded in your past and present. As if they are engaging with your traumas but also prophetic. It is unnerving. In poem after poem are expressions of grief over the loss of children, miscarriages, mental ill health, suicidal ideation and death. As if Eurydice had only ever been a mask, a costume to wear to let you perform, or prepare for, these experiences in disguise, and somehow I had failed to see so many of the connections at the time.

In 'The Drys' you write about a collective of *once and nearly mothers* gathered at a cliff edge where babies are *falling from the sky, shucked out from clouds*. A scene of desperate hands reaching and grasping as babies *snag and pulp […] on the harsh jut of my fingertips*. It is a nightmarish scene of mass maternal loss, a vision flung out of the body and into the world. In 'Hysteria' you write about a more intimate encounter, Eurydice remembering a miscarriage. *I felt an undoing – her/coming away/from my body's soft bite. Too soon.* It is the *too soon* that gets me now, the repeating double *oo*, the letters like the twins' first scan photo, the open-mouthed circular scream of those Os. Later the poem talks of *both of us sorting shadows*, which is exactly how it feels. Except your shadows are all I can access, the rest of you gone elsewhere. The *I* of the poem expresses how *the moorings of my body* [are] *loose*, an unleashing not only of physical but also mental matter. You are floating away from me but also away from yourself, and I feel there is nothing I can do to bring you back. Speaking of her transition from body to pure spirit your Eurydice writes, *It should be a mercy but now/my body's absence is solely/an echo chamber.*

The body is a site of memory, its gaps reminders of what was and what could have been, of the noise of all that feeling reverberating around the cavernous spaces. *Solely an echo chamber/waiting for music.* This seems to be where you are now, in this cave-like space, inside it, enveloped by it, it inside yourself. Waiting for that music of motherhood.

After weeks of vocalised anger you are now near-mute, too buried in it all to communicate how you are feeling. These poems feel like my way to make sense of some of it, even though they were written so many years before. Only now I see them in your mouth rather than Eurydice's. You are sinking into a depression, broken out of only by bouts of pain or anger. Your dad brushes your hair, but the act of care sees him accidentally pull too hard and the sharp shock of pain breaks you. The room is filled with a scream of rage from some deep volcanic well, from somewhere I don't recognise. You throw the brush at your dad with violent intent. When I hold you you feel different, unresponsive to touch, cold to it. When I look into your eyes you seem so far away, looking through me into another world all together.

In 'Host' you write, *Swans have settled/beneath my scalp,* then describe the way this flock of birds are wading through the circuitry of your brain, snagging and breaking the system, taking over. Mental illness as a form of violent colonisation. The poem ends with a beautiful threat, *This summer I walk carefully,/my brain full of eggs.* The sense of future chaos and damage having been implanted, waiting to hatch.

I've seen these patterns at various points over the last twelve years. It has come in waves before, sometimes triggered by a trauma and at other times harder to pin down. Sometimes you will be free of it for years, at other times we cling on to the months, weeks or even days when it seems to have faded or passed. You once called depression an *unmentionable weight*, and I have seen many times the ways it crushes you, sucks all the energy from your mind and body, straps you to the bed for days, builds walls between you and the outside world. I remember the early years in Cambridge when we would work so hard to muster the possibility of dragging you from bed for a short walk. Or the times anxiety has come, the constant alert and wait for a text or phone call, you breathless on the other end, holed up in a corner somewhere, a terrified animal version of yourself. Running, cycling, driving in panic to try and find you, to try and help you out of the mewling panic. In those moments it seems as if you are drowning in thin air. *Breathe*, I would say, over and over, as if it was the easiest thing in the world, a repeated mantra, hoping you will hear, hoping I can pull you from the depths. On these days I fear leaving you.

Perhaps it is no surprise that these poems from the past speak to your present. You had pointed me towards this in one of the poems when you wrote, *The wreck already had roots*, as if there was a grim reality to the destruction that depression and anxiety can cause, the paradox of burying a deep root system into the soil of self which means there is a future threat of it regrowing at any time.

You are sinking now to the kinds of places I have found you before, to the kinds of places where you might desire death over life. Your *Eurydice* poems are full of allusions to a desire for death. You speak of *drinking the dark/out of my own cupped hands*, depression itself as an elixir, a longing for a permanent darkness. In another poem you write, *My feet/root in mimicry of the slow ways/of a seed– I plant myself on a thin/scraping of dusk, waiting for the break/and spill*. It is a vision of her planting herself, of merely waiting for the moment in which she pours herself away into oblivion. When writing about Styx Eurydice states,

The river opens for me. You have always been drawn to water, in times of happiness and despair, and it seems to me that in these moments you would happily give yourself over to it, over to total and permanent forgetfulness.

In 'Learning to die' death *sounds like sleep*, is no more than a *long drop* with a *musical softness*. It is the softness of sleep that worries me, death seeming a release from the hard-edged world you are inhabiting: *breathing has a serrated edge,/and I must find means to separate from it.* You write of Eurydice meeting Persephone, the confrontation with a personification of death: *For a thin moment/I think she is my shadow.* We are used to distrusting the lyric *I* in poetry, we are used to understanding that the *I* of the poem's voice does not need to equate with the *I* of the poet, that it can be, and perhaps normally is, a different life that occupies the *I* of the poem. So when you wrote poems actively in the performative voice of a mythic character, then perhaps it was inevitable that I would acquit her of that *I* entirely. But here she is, here you are, echoing from the past of your own text, seeming to give voice and meaning to the things you cannot now express. You are speaking your future self through Eurydice's mouth.

Suicide is so often written about as a desperate and irrational act. Yet in recent literature there has been a pushback to this narrative. In *Notes on Suicide* Simon Critchley eruditely articulates how often suicide is a rational choice, a clear-eyed view of the choice of death being more appealing than the continuation of life. Without acknowledging this reality we have less chance of preventing people from getting to that point. If we cannot realise that to make that choice is rational, then we cannot untangle the suffocating problems that make someone feel that way. To suggest to someone who is suicidal that it is irrational is to push them, surely, closer to the edge. To acknowledge that the feelings have validity is, Critchley argues, the first step to helping them find a way to see life as more desirable than death. The alternative is hopelessness and nihilism, and with it the increased likelihood of someone acting on these feelings.

I have lived a good percentage of our relationship fearing you might take your own life. I remember seeing a flurry of texts and missed calls from our friend Daisy when I finished playing football one Friday night, rushing back to find you collapsed on the bathroom floor having overdosed on painkillers. I heard how you'd then panicked, called Daisy and made yourself sick to purge the pills. When I got there you were shaken, weak, as if the person who had taken the pills was your double, this figure of murderous intent lurking, stalking you, threatening you. The periods of suicidal thinking imprint themselves on future presents. It means that when you are not well I have to confront the possible risk that a text or call could come through that says you have done it. I have to let this possibility exist. To try and deny it would be to control your every move and to limit mine completely. It would be to freeze us both. I must not focus on the possible end but on trying to excavate the root systems beneath the wreck. Such gardening is a long and laborious digging in the dark.

I had learnt the ways to lift you out of darkness. Yet now I feel clueless and terrified. I can't fully comprehend the uniqueness of the connection between you and the pregnancies. I am a stranger in an alien land, with no sense of how to find you and bring you back. I keep thinking of the *thin ghosts* Ovid describes Orpheus passing through in the underworld. Here I am, stumbling in the dark passages, searching for what you are feeling, searching to find you, and only ever grasping at *thin ghosts*, at slippery shadows of your selfhood.

The studio started to feel frozen too. I was unable to paint. It all seemed pointless. Everything I had been trying to do felt neat and convenient, vacuous gestures at the connections between the paintings and what you were going through. I needed new ways in, ways to feel rather than to think towards new ways out. I had started to collect together the scraps from our previous Orpheus and Eurydice project. Your poems, filmed footage of performances and events, imagery from across the project. I needed to embed these pasts into the work, to use these words and images to open the work up further, and in doing so to find a way to reach and clasp towards you.

Some days, many days, I am paralysed by the fear. To see you vanish in increments is to be reminded of the possibility of your oblivion. I see you daily teetering at the edge, the possibility of you taking the leap hanging like a weather system in the house, in my head. Dark clouds gathering, like the encroaching arrival of thunder, oppressive and imminent. You are disappearing behind a curtain.

Blue had been the dominant colour of all the pre-fire Orpheus and Eurydice paintings, and in a number of the burnt canvases there were still flickers of its presence, or hints of it behind dark curtains of smoke-stained surfaces. It was an underworld built on the unstable foundations of blue. Stages, architecture, teeming masses of figures all moving through, on, and covered by great storms of blue paint. Blue was the colour of the voids from which one figure pulled another, blue was the sea and sky collapsing into and through rooms, blue was the colour of loss, of distance and mourning. Blue was the colour of entropy, the engine of chaos and dissolution.

It was a blue I had lifted from Titian, at first subconsciously and then with a manic embrace. It is a blue that appears through so many of his paintings and plays a dominant role in the *Poesie*

94

paintings, not just a representational signifier of sea or sky but always taking centre-stage in the drama of a viewer's encounter. Perhaps its most startling appearance is in his *Bacchus and Ariadne* (1523), one of three paintings Titian made for a scheme of mythological paintings for Alfonso d'Este. The commission, with various painters contributing mythological scenes inspired by poetic sources, serves as a kind of prototype of Titian's *Poesie* paintings.

It was the first painting I ever showed you. We were just officially together, but you were in the grips of a deep depression triggered by your assault in Cambridge a few months before. You had just given me a book of poems you had written in the long stretch of months at the start of our relationship, when I hadn't felt able to give you my heart. So when you asked me to show you some paintings it seemed the obvious choice. A painting of a poem. A painting as a poem.

The painting's source is the mythological subject matter from poems by Ovid and Catullus. The bottom right-hand half is overspilling with Bacchus and his entourage, returning from their triumph in India. On the far left is Ariadne, recently abandoned by her lover Theseus on the island of Naxos. Bacchus leaps, desire-bound, across the painting's central divide, towards Ariadne, his motion echoed by a curved, windswept coral-coloured fabric. The impending union will be an embrace in which the god transforms the mortal Ariadne into a constellation of stars.

Blue is the thread that stiches these narrative episodes into one frame. Ariadne is draped in a blue robe, which sculpts and echoes the corkscrew motions of her entire body. She is in the motion of turning from facing outwards towards the horizon, to the site of Theseus' boat, which is on course to vanish off the left-hand edge of the picture frame, then caught by the surprise air-bound arrival of Bacchus. Her body is moving not just through space, but through narrative time and psychological consequence. The body records these movements and the blue of her robe functions beyond decoration and motion. It locates blue, in this instance, as the solidity of corporeal presence, but which reaches towards the shifting sands of multitudes. Behind her, the sea and the sky, both wide stretches of the same blue, its tone shifted, lighter, spread out. The sea is the stage of Theseus' departure, the deep waters of the past carrying the depths and weight of mourning. In contrast, the huge expanse of sky, with the crown of stars, the eternal future awaiting Ariadne, the endless, weightless space of the eternal.

Ariadne's hand is still turned out towards the horizon. Turned flat, as if waving, but also seeming to press towards the vast space, as if it might be able to push up against the endless distance, so pressed longingly into a void, into the blue.

As Bogdan Wolf notes, blue is *detached from its purely representational function*. Here blue holds a vast spectrum of narrative and psychological functions. For the viewer it becomes our entry point, it becomes the wide-open space to fall into, to feel into. It also spills into us, an endlessly wide sky of eternity, the impossible deep sea of mourning, the twisting cloth of our spin through time and space. Perhaps that hand does not reach out, as Bogdan Wolf contemplates, but attempts to hold off the sudden flood of the colour that covers half of the canvas and threatens to drown us. Blue as the site of our oblivion.

The same blue appears in the sky and in the dress of the Mary in Titian's *Pesaro Madonna* (1519–26), which he was working on before, during and after *Bacchus and Ariadne*. His wife Cecilia posed for the figure of Mary, holding the wriggling baby Jesus. They had just married (1525) and would have three children, before Cecilia died in childbirth in 1530. In *Bacchus and Ariadne* we see Titian's ability to flood a colour with psychological weight. Now the blue of oblivion pours out of the painting, floods into his life. And as if projecting backwards, narcissistically, I now can't see that blue and not fear a similar form of loss, the limitless depth of a feared-for grief.

That seeping, flooding, again, the same blue running through my sense of you. To the past, to you standing in front of *Bacchus and Ariadne* as I waffle on, seeing you connect so specifically and deeply to the blue as if it was poured into you as pure feeling. Then blue in your *Eurydice* poems over a decade later. The first of which opens: *Let's start with the sky yes the sky the sky/that day was all sorts of blue.* Like in the paintings, an entire underworld, a selfhood, the past and present all overflowing with blue, whether it be seas, skies, boats or the *blue dark* you speak of occupying. Blue as the colour of your entire inner world. Now again, with the threat of your suicide hanging like a heavy cloud, threatening to spill out of the skies and oceans of your oblivion.

It is a painting of beautiful oblivion that generates a small flicker of light in you. Jadé Fadojutimi had produced three huge canvases for the Venice Biennale. Like many of her works, they carry, and are propelled forwards by, enigmatic titles: *The Prolific Beauty of Our Panicked Landscape*; *And that day, she remembered how to purr*; and *Rebirth*. We had just cancelled a third planned research trip to Venice, the first two due to Covid, the most recent due to your recovery. I had showed you these three paintings on my laptop, mediated through the backlit glow of the computer. The screen, so often a distancing device in engaging with a painting, seemed to offer you a hope of something. You have been existing in the perpetual present, one enveloped by your suicidal ideations. Somehow, viewing these paintings together in the dark of night from our bed acts as a kind of transportation, the glow of a possible future, of another place, of an escape from the self and the now.

All three of the paintings entrance us, but it is *The Prolific Beauty of Our Panicked Landscape* that seems to send you into a kind of trance. For the first time in so long I see a pulse of recognition, a flicker of life in your eyes, as if a sliver of you is returning, or offering the hope of return. I cling to this moment, to the painting as an agent of ignition, the lighting of a small glimmer flame of light in the dark.

Even on the small screen the painting feels as if it is the size of a cinema screen, as if it holds a power which refuses to be shrunk and flattened by the normal deadening translation of digital reproduction. The canvas is full of an extraordinary array of vibrant colours and lively marks, but they all sit within or behind great vertical drags of translucent umber. It reads like a thin curtain, creating the effect of light pouring through it, bringing the array of other marks, colours and movements into a unity, into an interplay with this painted sheet of textile and light. The way the light seems to flood through this translucent sheet of paint recalls sun pouring in through the curtains of a bedroom window or stained-glass.

The rest of the marks lead us into a grand dance. There is a neon-pink thick outline of a triangle, brightly coloured hand-painted circles, the wobble of imprecision giving them movement, like cells floating and pulsing. Other shapes suggest nature, flowers or petals or the branch of a tree, but with high saturations. Daubs of paint, shapes without clear reference, gather in clusters like the tracked motion and layering of forms of leaves in autumn. Everywhere there is the sense of the hand, or the body having been present, not through image or indexical marks but just through the motioning of the lines, through the fluidity of movement, through the haptic sense in which the pressure has varied and been interrupted by the rhythm of the body's motions.

Fadojutimi's studio is set up like a stage, where all the parts are players. The canvases are both smaller stages within this set-up, awaiting the action of painting, and actors in the unfolding and interconnected drama, from which the paintings both emerge and feed back into. Everything in the studio is arranged in a careful and conscious curation. The objects she chooses to surround herself with – plants, chairs, teddies – are not just for decoration, comfort or function, but integral parts of the machinery she uses to create the paintings.

Some of the teddy bears are old, fragile companions from childhood. Stitched together, full of holes, the material of the things barely holding. Such attachments to the past, to nostalgia, form sources of emotional substance for her to pull from and flush into her paintings. She talks of crying while painting, she embraces being earnest, she allows the work to come from within her, in a way that can too easily be dismissed as anachronistic or the mythologising of romanticism. As if we can outgrow deep and honest feeling. She writes, *I am always happy to shed enough tears, to fill every pocket as a painting.*

Writing plays an important role in her work, and not just in the enigmatic titles she gives the paintings. In a publication about her work by Anomie Press and Pippy Houldsworth Gallery, passages of her poetic texts sit on coloured translucent sheets, layered over reproductions of whole paintings or details of surfaces. This palimpsest sets up an ekphrastic relationship between the text and the image, but one can then be pulled back to see the painting alone.

The familiar is as ripe a hunting ground for Fadojutimi as the things she draws from her travels. Her long love affair with Japan is a central influence. Her paintings gather together the strange and the familiar, the new and the old, the past and the present as if they are equal companions on a journey into uncanny lands.

She is interested in what she calls the *Elasticity of imagination within limits of familiar walls*; the ways in which the everyday, even the seemingly mundane, can become the source material of an ever-expanding universe.

What does an eye that devours everything make of a world full of darkness? The paintings in Venice were made during Covid, and at the same time as the Black Lives Matter protests. Fadojutimi writes about the pressures and expectations put upon her, as a young Black woman making work within this climate and context:

At times, my imagination has been taken and my freedom stolen. I've spent countless times being forced to imagine things like equality, I spend my time imagining people not having to die to live. I can only imagine a world without racial prejudice. I have to spend more time imagining ways of living that are unknown realities to me.

I can't breathe became the refrain of the Black Lives Matter movement in the United States. It was the repeated utterance of Eric Garner as he was murdered by the chokehold of a New York City police office in 2014. To see a young artist pressured into politicising her work is to see breath taken again. This pressure is a form of structural racism where the freedoms afforded others are not so easily afforded to Black artists, who should not be chained to geopolitical and historical struggles that others have decided should be their chief concern.

Fadojutimi writes about how she is *desperate to catch every breath*, how she wants to pour so much energy and feeling into her paintings that *now my paintings will just breathe*. She seems to approach life and painting with a passionate need to fill her lungs, her body and her paintings with all the wonders of the world.

At one point I began inhaling as much as I could, as
though I had wasted so much time not breathing
before
… But now I want to gulp down this tedious time called
life, perhaps just to choke
on the excitement, who knows?

She writes about the imagination being a tool to expand the world, *not hold us in place*, because *living is truly remarkable*. She sees no boundaries between the different aspects of her life, which feed each other. She is alive to the world, and makes us alive to it as well.

Her artistic process is energetic and at times close to a dance with the canvas. She is often led by intuition, by the directions opened up by initially instinctive marks. Using Liquin, a high-gloss medium which thins down acrylics, her paint moves fluidly across the surface and provides a semi-transparency that characterises many of her marks. Oil sticks are used for drawn lines of paint which meander across the surface, picking up wet layers and confusing the distinctions between the different depths and layers. Sometimes the paintings are knotted and tight and tense, but the Venice paintings seem to open up. She says, *they become environments for me. They reflect myself and they become spaces for me to exist. To be born into.* They are also environments for the viewer. They are grand, cinematic landscapes. As she states:

I'm constantly walking along the edge of a cliff afraid
To be blown over at the instant of a slight breeze

We walk this tightrope with her in *The Prolific Beauty of Our Panicked Landscape*, a painting which seems posed in tension. The impressions of hands and bodies are everywhere. Three purple arrangements of lines read like huge arrows, pointing us in all directions including down towards the edge, to the threshold of the picture plane. The arrows seem to say 'Enter here', 'Exit there', as if pulling us in and pushing us back out in a fluid and continuous cycle. There are great washes and stains of colours from the luminous yellows and orange of the top left-hand corner, which read like a child's depiction of an exploded sun painted in highlighter pen. To the right is a pale-purple stain, as if everything in the painting is dissolving, or taking shape.

Perhaps the three arrows signify the artist, the viewer, the body, the hand and then the eye moving across this edge, the arrows both a direction of movement and a warning. The thin curtain suggests that we are simultaneously inside and outside, on both sides of a window, or even locked in the pane itself, looking both ways. The cliff edge brought into the bedroom, the great vast drop the edge of the bed. Then we are in a dream space at that point of being just about to fall, or falling, but not falling into sleep, an infinite yet non-existent depth sculpted by the limitless physics of the mind.

Fadojutimi talks of her studio recreating the conditions of her bedroom, building safety and the known into her practice. She wants her paintings to emerge from the place where dreams happen and memories are formed, and where we rest. She dissolves the distinction between the work and domestic space. In *The Prolific Beauty of Our Panicked Landscape* a waking dream is made solid. It captures the meeting point between two realms. Perhaps we see each other in her paintings, or perhaps we just feel the gust of wind left by a ghost. We sense a figure who was there at another time, and for just a moment our eyes reach as hands through the curtained border.

Fadojutimi cites great colourists as influences, such as Lee

Under

Krasner, Henri Matisse, Joan Mitchell and Amy Sillman, a host of artists for whom colour was feeling, a way into the world and life. Standing in front of *The Prolific Beauty of Our Panicked Landscape* I feel like the wanderer in Friedrichs' iconic romantic landscape. But in Fadojutimi's work the protagonist is outside the landscape, the painting the scene. A great sea of fog fills with a dance of abstract marks that record a kaleidoscopic history of painting, swirling like the Northern Lights. I see within her work a constellation of painters for whom paint was a poetic language, with colour as its driver. But her work is never pastiche or ironic. The landscape of the painting is built on so many visual stimuli. We are maybe floating, flying, rising. Existing in a space free of singular gravity, unleashed from earthly and bodily limits, transcending into pure feeling.

This unadulterated intense feeling is felt through the body, flows on and into the canvas, and then back again. As she writes, *I want my gut to roll around in paint so it can colour and smear my soul as I sing*, later calling painting *a gushing experience*. Sensations flow like great geysers of fluid, or orgiastic ejaculations across the canvas.

I love to swell
I love to push past my tummy in order for it to spread

There is a sensual energy to the connection, imagery which stretches and swells, is rushed through with blood and desire like the lust-filled workings of a body:

For me, love was flowing into my paintings like a river

Perhaps this sensuality is awoken in you when you view the paintings on the screen. You had been detached from the world and from your body. Something in these paintings prompts a reawakening, a kinaesthetic response.

One of the three vast canvases Jadé Fadojutimi made for the Venice Biennale was titled *Rebirth*. Dominated by the backdrop of lush, vibrant greens, the bottom edge has a wave of red, a divide between the viewer and the verdant distance. Rebirth suggests not just an arrival into life, but an arrival into life from death – the exact movement that Eurydice desired. Viewing this painting, we are enlivened, brought back in touch with the richness of life, brought into contact with the motions of beauty itself.

Yet the flicker of recognition that you feel is temporary. You sink back further into yourself. I wonder about the possibility of making paintings, of staging something that might reignite this feeling in you. I need to work harder to find you, to pull you back. I am losing you.

The studio feels like a site of possible retrieval. I decide to take your poems as prompts for a performance, to move language into action, and words into image. I will use the paintings I had been making and the burnt detritus from the previous Orpheus and Eurydice project as my props for an improvisation.

I wanted to bridge the space between you and me.

I build a set of an underworld. I start by arranging the studio into a theatrical stage, clearing out the centre so that it is a blank space awaiting action. At the back I have all the materials piled up. A camera is set up in the corner, raised to give a voyeuristic view of the action. I set it to record. I rehang one of the unstretched canvases, walk up to it, reach out to touch the surface, and then repeat the motion from a variety of angles. I'm thinking about touch and distance, about the depths in the canvas that are beyond the material limits. In your poem 'Sapling' you write about Eurydice pressing *with a single finger pushed through shade/Root-struck, scanning for sun.* A figure buried in the earth, pushing back up to the surface. As you write later in the poem, *it is only at a distance/this place holds any shape*, while to be in it, or to be at the border of it, is to see the formlessness of the space and the life within it.

I think about the hanging canvas as the divide. I step around it, my body disappearing from the view of the camera lens. A foot or arm is visible at the edges. Orpheus steps into the underworld, through to the hidden space behind the painting, behind the veil and screen. I turn, look back at the canvas from the other side, am unseen by the camera. My feet beneath are the only visible sign of presence, of a body facing back towards us. Could these feet now be Eurydice's returning from the underworld, vanishing back into it? I am trying to capture the act of appearance and disappearance. I reverse the actions and enact the process of appearing, of returning to the other side of the canvas, crossing from the hidden realm to the seen world. I do it over and over, to get as much coverage as possible. In 'Form' you write, *You came quietly through trees/to make me human.* I hang multiple canvases, repeat the motion of walking into them, through them, back through them. The figure is only ever caught in glimpses or in the process of becoming a glimpse; a thin ghost.

I meditate on the line *to make me human.* It resonates with the myth of Eurydice but also with the pregnancies, our babies stolen from us. I think of the surgery and of possible life trapped in a tube, arrested in its journeying into being. What is it in painting and in pregnancy, for one human to make another?

I strip the canvases from the ceiling and lay them in a stack on the floor. I undress and wrap one of the large sheets of painted fabric around me as a rudimentary costume, a cloak covering me. I walk in it, let it cocoon me, only one hand, two feet and a glimpse of face in the shadow. I shift the head to let an eye or a mouth be revealed to the view of the camera, appearing from the dark. I cover myself entirely and lie down on the floor, the body now sculpting the fabric from within, becoming something other than human, something hidden. I play with letting one limb, a foot or hand, appear at the edge, as if a buried body, or a hand with the palm turned up, is pleading for the viewer's returning palm. The image is now a living sculpture, a form shifting in the studio. There is a hole in the studio floor which had been used many years ago as a mechanics pit. I lay canvas flat over the hole, then climb down and into it. I record this figure vanishing into the buried space beneath the floor.

Looking at the footage on the camera, it feels too flat. I want to complicate and confuse the space in the frame. The studio is now stacked with canvases on stretcher bars, with other burnt paintings where the canvas hangs off the brittle black framework. There are stacks of loose burnt bars on the floor and empty stretcher frames. From this detritus of the previous Orpheus and Eurydice project I build the new underworld. Paintings lean against each other, canvases drop over the top, frames stack up vertically. Clumsy cuboid forms, half collapsed, just held together, purposefully precarious, like a sculptural sketch of an early cubist painting. These are stage sets awaiting the arrival of a protagonist. The camera is set up again, the angle occasionally varied, the body of material covering many hours over the days and weeks.

I repeat similar actions of entering and exiting. I find points in the structure that might read like a window, or a door. I pull back fabrics and reach through, or pull them back from the inside to reveal a face or a limb. I pull the structure down on top of me, let myself become buried in it and then rebuild. Inside the structure I roll, fling myself up to allow a leg to emerge, the last vignette of a falling body into it. A naked body in a slow dance with the static architecture.

In your 'Chorus' poems the underworld itself seemed to speak in musical rhythms: *in a backward glance it will all come down crashing her/face a night-lit smudge something rising through darkness/a moon silent and cratered the o of her lips caught/forever on the tide of his eyes.* It was this backward glance I was trying to enact, a moment when everything crashed down and collapsed in on itself. I wanted to capture the violence and destructive energy and the implosion of space that the glance and the gaze caused.

I want to become the subject and the object, to absent myself from the normal responsibilities, coordinates and power of the self. The camera is the passive, non-sentient observer, whose position and perspective are purposefully limited. I want to be, for a brief moment, occupying the hidden space of the gaze itself. That *night-lit smudge* rising from the darkness, the *o of her lips caught/forever on the tide of his eyes.* There in the shadows the vanishing form of you gives a last gasped breath of an O, a silent mouth shaped into an ambivalent mixture of pain and ecstasy.

The performances are theatrical events without an audience. The witnessing is deferred while the camera captures footage for a possible future viewer. My desires are numerous: I want to act out something similar to the state of the painting, where the viewer is absent from the performance, only able to access the aftermath. I want to step outside the role of artist and become a participant in the drama of the painting itself. I want to step outside myself in order to look back at the footage with the fresh eyes of the viewer. I want I want I want. I become possessed by the process and the world opened up by it. It is as much about what the camera can't capture as what I will take forward.

I view the footage on the camera and select the best clips,

arranging them into a crudely collaged film. The studio is rearranged again, another combination of the frames, canvases and veiling fabrics. I set up a projector and cast the film footage across the space, so that it is scattered across a number of the angled surfaces of the rudimentary staged structure. The projection is both a stage light and a generator of imagery, which is chucked across canvases, vanishing at borders, into the dark. On white surfaces the imagery is sharp, on the painted canvases it blends, appearing to be embedded within them. The imagery animates the paintings, as if it is moving from the paint itself. Elsewhere frames of the burnt canvases throw shadows cutting the shape of a sitting-room window across the wall and floor.

When I enter the stage, the imagery falls on my body. My face is expanded across a screen. I reach out to touch it, before the figure retreats into the optical distance. Elsewhere a body is broken, legs appearing, the rest lost to the opening of the frame, dissolved into the darkness of the distance presented. The projected images are not clear cinematic footage. Broken up and confused, they are like disordered memory traces. In Eurydice's voice you had written, *now my body's/absence is solely an echo chamber/waiting for music.* I was trying to build this echo chamber and for it to resonate with absences.

Looking back at the new footage, the body seems too normalised, too real compared to the language that is developing in the rest of the space. It needs to be made of the stuff of the underworld. Painting begins with a primed canvas, so I prepare my body, covering it in white paint and thinned-down clay. It is a second skin, as if I am half vanished or masked, inside something else. The slick, viscous mixture slowly congeals, first slipping across and then clinging to the body. A body broken from the limits of my appearance and identity.

This second skin liberates the performance, injecting it with a new energy. I climb, fall through, and fling myself across the stage set, often collapsing it and then rebuilding again, body bruised, skin needing a fresh covering of paint and clay. I look to the edges, to the borders, be that where the imagery breaks across a surface or the edge of a canvas on the floor, or the entrance into the structure. My actions are focused on crossing these barriers. The figure, it occurs to me, is in search of something. It is mourning, longing.

The projected imagery sings on the body, a previous version of me moving itself across my skin, the space of the studio drawing sharp lines and grids on to the torso. The performance, the filmed footage and the painting, is a self-generating mutating machine. An underworld which forms itself in a constant feedback loop, expanding and deepening, creating its own rules of engagement.

I was trying to reach the empty space between you and me, between any two bodies, be that between lovers, the painter and the painting, or the viewer and the artwork, even the primal relationship between you and the lost babies to be. I wanted to walk towards that gap in the hope that I might be able to see it, feel it, paint it.

I thought of you, and the wholeness of you. In the Eurydice poems you say, *I wasn't some slick girl/dropping her skin by the water's edge … I wasn't a hooked fish/pinned and gasping on the slats/while a man steadies his knife.* The lover can't be possessed as mere image and body, violently cut or sliced out of the world, reduced to a flattened form. Later you wrote, *I was a blue dark/ long before I met you,* Eurydice saying that Orpheus – *came too late to my body/to know – /the wreck already had roots.* Your histories and selfhood are wider and deeper than the limits of your knowledge.

I would be lying if I told you that the artwork I was creating was all about you. I didn't have enough control over it or knowledge of or possession of it. It was beyond me and the limits of the studio, and had a life of its own. It contained shadows from sources I had not created. Viewed on film, it is an uncomfortable world to look at. It reads as a crypt containing deeply buried forms of memory and trauma, a walled-off space accidentally stumbled upon. What is seen there? What is heard there? Where did it come from? Where is it going?

When I think of your possible death, I am weighed down by a grief without limits. Perhaps I am in the studio searching in three directions: towards the fear of that possible future, the state of anxiety in the present, and the relation of all this to the deeply buried roots of your past. The material generated by days and weeks of working in the studio grows exponentially, while in contrast you are locked in stasis. Your stitches are now fully healed, you are mobile again and pain-free, but you have *dropped your skin at the water's edge.* You have *entered the blue dark*, and I can't work how to pull you out. I feel sadness for the loss of our babies, but abject terror of losing you.

7

Embrace

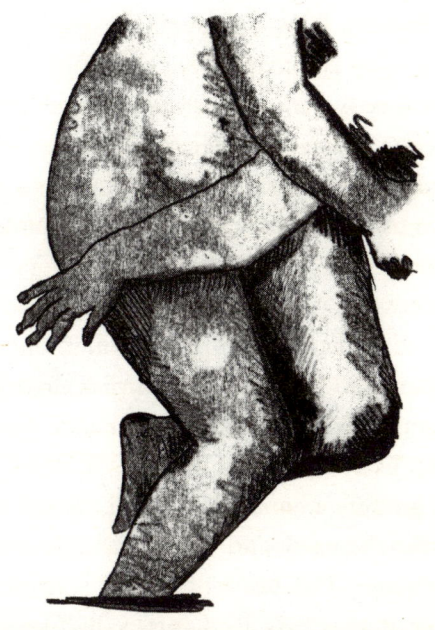

I cling to certainty when we wake up in the morning, your leg over mine. You are still here. Some mornings I wake and there is a space where you were, my arm across cool sheets. I fear the worst. These mornings I call out and your voice calls back. You climb into bed and we curl into each other, and I wonder if perhaps it is possible to never let go.

In Ovid's *Metamorphoses*, Book X, Orpheus sings the song of

Venus and Adonis. This is how Adonis was born: in the trunk of a tree a womb swells, the tree bending its heavy branches to the ground, weeping a shower of leaves to the floor. A deep groan, a creak and crack as the trunk splits open, the skin of bark exposing an opening from which the child falls. Although he was already fallen, conceived in sin, fated to die as a result of his mortal urges, he is born into the world an enviable beauty.

Years are slippery, falling through the gaps of a single line of poetry. The baby is a man, more beautiful than ever, and a hunter. His beauty is a magnet, attracting the desire and then the love of Venus. Love pulls her from Heaven, and in a tight embrace she offers up her warning and her fears – to not be foolish in his drive to hunt. She leaves him, sky-bound in a chariot pulled by swans.

Adonis ignores the warnings and his dogs nose a boar. Soon the hunter is the hunted, running now, till in one mighty blow his motion is arrested by the bloodied tusk driven through his groin. Left dying, bleeding out, into the earth. The last breaths of life reach up to Venus. Spinning, she descends, full of grief and rage. She gathers a handful of blood, makes a potion of it, spills it back into the earth and watches as a deep-red anemone sprouts and blooms. The burst of beauty is brief, a gust stripping the flower of its petals. Red curves, half-hearts, dispersed on the wind.

How to picture all of this? Titian does it with an embrace. He made a number of copies of his *Venus and Adonis* painting, but documentary evidence suggests that the version in the Prado is the one he sent to Philip II as part of the *Poesie* cycle. Space is used to organise time. On the left, in mid-distance, Cupid lies in shaded slumber beneath the canopy of a tree. Here is the past, love's work done. On the right, in deeper distance, is the clustering of trees, the edge of a forest which spreads out beyond the frame. A beam of light shines down from the breaking clouds, from which a shimmering suggestion of Venus on her chariot appears. Here lies the future, and Adonis' death. In the foreground Venus holds Adonis in a loving, desperate embrace. The movements of their bodies contain narration.

Venus is naked, sitting on a rock covered with a rich, soft purple fabric. She has her back turned to us, the top and bottom of her body a corkscrew of opposing forces, which communicate the dramatic shift on the scene. The bottom half sees her legs open, facing the back and left of the picture frame. Her torso twists towards the right, her arms reaching to enclose Adonis. The animation of the body and the counter-forces of its two halves articulate the shift, from the stasis of the embrace to the desperate desire to cling on. Adonis mirrors this. His torso is still turned towards Venus, still facing each other, eyes locked. He leans forwards, right leg bent in motion, body crossing the halfway points of the painting's vertical and horizontal axis. Both bodies and the picture's composition depict a struggle, between Venus' desire and Adonis' mortal urge to hunt. The drama of Ovid's tragedy is captured within the dynamics of this embrace.

The embrace contains a fear of absence, both temporary and permanent. What might it look like to paint figures, bodies and forces which express not the potential of this absence but its presence? What would it be to picture the isolated figure, when the other is merely memory? What if the forces of the other on our body remain, but their body is gone?

Due to the number of losses, we are placed into a cycle of testing. The recurrent miscarriage clinic, run by a top fertility consultant, begins what feels like a detective investigation. They take our bloods time and again, to rule things out as much as diagnose. They do a series of endometrial scratches, scans and what seems like constant prodding and poking. On one occasion we are both in the same clinic to give samples. You are taken away for bloods while I am shown to a strange little cubicle to produce the sperm sample. There is a small hatch which opens for me to place the sample in, before closing it and pressing a button to let the invisible humans the other side collect it. I wait for you in the cavernous glass reception, toy with screaming at the top of my lungs.

Bit by bit they are able to tell us what the problem isn't. It becomes increasingly clear that they can't locate a specific cause, and therefore cannot offer a possible solution. We become amateur researchers, spending our evenings reading books, journal articles and going down dangerous Google holes in a desperate search for answers. We make lists of questions to ask at every appointment, go through all the results of tests looking for a sign of something.

Eventually you are diagnosed with hyperfertility. It is a catch-all term to describe a series of conditions where the endometrium appears to be especially receptive to implantation. It means that even non-viable embryos – a term we come to detest – implant, as the lining of the womb is not able to distinguish between the 'quality' of each embryo. There is less than ten years of concrete research on the condition, meaning there are more unknowns than knowns. An online article describes early research which shows the cells in the womb-lining of women with hyperfertility to be *reaching out to all kinds of embryos*. Cells reach out and cling on to embryos destined to not survive. I have no idea how scientifically accurate the description is, whether cells do reach out in the process of implantation, as opposed to just receive, but the personification resonates. The cellular structure of your womb seems to be mirroring the desperate desire we have, to reach out, to hold on to the possibilities presented by each pregnancy. The literature around hyperfertility describes it as a theoretical condition, partly because it is often diagnosed through a process of elimination and partly because there is still so little known about it. Even the diagnosis of a condition is surrounded by the possibility of it not existing. The language of medicine matters, and this phrase *a theoretical condition* cuts through. We now have a diagnosis that the literature is not even able to confirm exists.

In our attempt to find out as much as possible about the condition we stumble across its more colloquial use, where it seems to be applied, without medical validity, to describe the supposed hyperfertility of various ethnic groups. In one demoralising Zoom with a fertility specialist who rules out IVF, he asked about your heritage. When you tell him you are quarter Indian, on your mum's side, he nods in a patronising manner, and as casually as anything says, yes, that could be it, South Asians often have a higher rate of fertility. We initially take it for granted, but after doing some research we discover that he is conflating the new studies around hyperfertility as a medical condition with hyperfertility as a term used to project spurious claims about various ethnicities being more fertile. It is an area of sociological research that behavioural and data scientists such as Dr Pragya Agarwal have extensively explored. Her research considers the unconscious biases that the medical profession projects on to women from certain backgrounds struggling with fertility. This particular doctor was merging an unscientific sociological presumption with biological concerns. Both the original premise and the connection between the two are unfounded. At the end of the call, having said there was nothing he could to do help he signed off, *have you thought about trying to lose some weight*. Not only was the delivery insensitive and offhand, it wasn't based in the specifics of our situation. We'd been told by the main specialist that the loss of the babies was categorically nothing to do with weight. When we sign out from Zoom, in place of the anger I expect to see, you are ashen, sucked of all energy. You feel failed by your body and failed by the experts we are putting our hopes in. Fury rumbles inside me – at the circumstances, but more directly at this arrogant man. His behaviour is the antipathy of a being a good doctor, where scientific expertise and an understanding of the human experience should meet.

He had ruled out several paths, including IVF, because our issue was not getting pregnant but staying pregnant. Along with his other comments he suggested that we should be fine if we *just keep trying. It would work eventually.* As if the losses had no cost, as if it was merely a case of rolling the dice until the right numbers came up. It struck me that he had no comprehension, and made no attempt to imagine into, what it must feel like to carry and then lose a baby. How those losses are utterly exhausting, physically and psychologically, however early they happen. What he saw as hope we felt as hopelessness. We were being sent out into the dark with the knowledge that we would likely continue to have more losses. Luckily the specialist we are under has deep reservoirs of empathy, despite being over-worked and stretched to breaking point. She guides us gently, with a care in her communication and a humility in explaining what she knows and where the gaps are. She makes us feel like partners in the process, and her approach is collaborative. Her small gestures are lights helping us to step again into the dark.

We try again and you are pregnant again. The appearance of the line on the test no longer brings joy but fills us with fear. We wait, and day by day we let hope sneak back in, drop by drop.

It is uncanny that you constructed your mythology of Eurydice around the idea of multiple miscarriages. The poems pre-empted what has followed. They gave voice to what is now happening. Your poem 'Hysteria' is one of waiting. It opens with the body's loosening ties. *I felt an undoing – her/coming away/from my body's soft bite.* That phrase, *soft bite*, the tender violence of it, the way it now mirrors what has been happening in your womb. The cells reaching out and holding on, the *soft bite* of that desire, the *undoing* and *coming away*. The poem ends with the arrival of the loss, *the moorings of [your] body* coming loose, and then the final line, isolated in its own white space ...

(just starting to bleed)

The centre of the poem exists in a liminal space. It describes Eurydice walking in the early hours along a riverbank, settling to watch *a heron stoop in the shallows,/scanning/for the silver shift/for an arrival.* The figure is in something close to a dream and the heron might be a metaphor of the psyche, searching for life to either emerge or be pulled from the mirrored surface of the river. This is the hysteria you are alluding to in the title, as opposed to the pain of the loss that sandwiches this scene. The hysteria of waiting, the moments when you can still hold hope. Hysteria could untether itself at any moment, could be released from your grasp. We are there now, scanning the surface, not quite in the real world, but somewhere along this riverbed searching for that fish.

Then it happens again. The knotting in the stomach and the bleeding. Another loss. You seem to be going further in, beyond the shallows, into deeper water, further from land, further from me. You are inside yourself, separating from the world.

It sounds strange to say we are haunted by the losses, but in a very matter-of-fact way we are. Across these years there are babies born to friends and family. Dissonance is the word for the hauntings. We can be with friends or family and I see it in your eyes, see you looking at another baby playing, knowing that you are imagining one of our would-be, could-have-been children alongside them. We see the tired eyes of other new parents and long for that tiredness, which we once dreaded. Then time shifts and the babies become toddlers. The haunting doesn't pass, and at these moments we see little shadow toddlers wearing our faces, little ghosts alone next to the others.

In all my fears of you taking your life I had seen it as a binary, either you would live or die. Those were the options. Yet there is something else happening here. You are becoming spectral. I catch you in moments during the joy and flow of a group setting when I suspect you have been haunted by our unborn little ones wandering up from the underworld, and you are a ghost, only half here, semi-faded from the world. I wonder if in this spectral state you can, perhaps, even briefly, touch them. I wonder if they will ever leave us, whether we even want that. I wonder whether you will ever truly come back. It strikes me that my construction of the underworld in the studio is wrong. You are Orpheus as much as you are Eurydice. You are searching in the underworld for your lost loves, wanting to bring them back, knowing that you can't.

Running through the centre of your Eurydice poems is a chorus, written from the perspective of the witness figures in the underworld. The lines flow into each other, as if the poem has a voice that comes from many bodies and that runs in one long, desperate breath. There is a passage which seems to capture the unwieldy nature of things you are now feeling, of the way everything seems to be happening to you, all control taken, even over your own body:

when will they learn the shape of things stop it
has a fearful momentum they must stop it
will not come good in the end no way to stop it
now monsters are coming look down yes down

The three-fold repeat of *stop it* at the end of each line expresses a desire to halt the momentum of not just the poem but the inevitability of what is to follow. Monsters are coming, racing up behind the shadows which seem to be chasing everything forwards. There is a dizzying quality to the downward gaze, the sense that everything could tumble down at any moment, back into the underworld and its monsters.

But what are the monsters? You are having increasingly toxic and monstrous thoughts, and I'm worried you are mistaking the thoughts for facts. We are starting to drift, alienated from each other, however much we try to stay connected. You have nowhere to put these thoughts and I am incapable of holding them for you, so they fester, seed and sink in their roots. The distance between us grows with unforeseen scale and force, an invisible barrier expanding exponentially between us. You stop telling me what you are thinking, say that your thoughts are unspeakable or unsayable.

We are faced with the uncomfortable reality that our desire to have a child is something we are unable to switch off, whatever the pain trying to have one will cause. I wonder if there is a danger that we are conditioned to think it is a choice, that in having decided it is what we want we are programmed to just keep chasing, an unrelenting pursuit that we will continue until it breaks us. I am starting to resent the attempts, the pregnancies, the losses. I hate what it is doing to you, the way it is slowly ripping you, and us, apart. I want us to stop the inevitability that we will keep trying. I want us to let go of the idea of having a child, as if that would be the easiest thing in the world. I know you can't, and I'm not sure, if push came to shove, I could either. I am terrified of it all.

In the graphic novel we made together the underworld was full of the monsters your poem mentions. It was an underworld overflowing with a vast population of creatures. Sometimes whole seas would be crammed with boats full, or entire skies patterned with them. They lurked in forests, came screaming out of shattered and angular mirrors, morphed into shadows across walls or spiralled outwards into vast labyrinthine architectures. They were everywhere.

When I thought of you as both Orpheus and Eurydice, wandering the underworld of your own body, I wondered what monsters you were seeing. I tried to picture them, thought about painting them. Yet these are the scariest monsters, the monsters who exist beneath the bed, the monsters who only show you their shadow or a single claw. In the gaps of our imagination we create our worst nightmares, populating the darkness with possibilities which stretch beyond the seen. You are now wandering the voids left by their various departures, just able to access the spaces they leave behind.

The 2021 film *The Rescue* documents the Tham Luang cave rescue, when in 2018 a young Thai football team got trapped in an underground cave system due to rising water levels. As the rain continued, the water levels rose and the acoustics of the space were altered. Underground, in this network of caves, with many passages submerged, sound no longer sculpted space in the same way. Everything was dispersed, abstracted, the form and origin of sound impossible to locate. The noises reverberated around and through the interior walls, coming from everywhere and nowhere. I picture the underworld you inhabit now, the one inside you, as something akin to this. The body is a system of submerged caves, each loss a part of the body opened up, hollowed out, carved in stone. You are wandering, swimming, struggling for breath. The sounds of the past few years, all those voices, echoing through, separating themselves from the bodies from which they came, arriving as the disturbed un-locatable voices of the monsters in the dark.

Every day in my imagination I enter the room to find you there, having taken your life. This thought sits like a ghost on my shoulder, and I have to accept it as possible. It only vanishes in the moment I see you and touch you again. Every day I lose you in my mind. When Orpheus watched Eurydice fall back into the underworld, to die a second time, it was to realise that his vision was murderous. He saw her vanish, again, watched her disappear into death. I'm grieving your possible death, suspended and held. I am watching you fall again and again, but sight heals, and to see you is to know you are still here. Even in the moments where death seems unlikely, like a fear I can soften, I am still watching you fade. I am losing you to one underworld or another. I am reaching out but I cannot touch you.

It is strange to grieve something that has not gone.

My studio has become a self-perpetuating archive. I have been printing off hundreds of images from my performances, film stills and photographs. Everywhere there are images of figures entering spaces, falling, reaching, half hidden, veiled or multiplied across various surfaces. I've been collecting up photographs of you, from across the thirteen years of our relationship, keen to access something of the unstaged naturalism of them. There are also hundreds of photographs of the two of us poised for the Orpheus and Eurydice project, of us lifting, dragging or embracing the other, the force of one body exerted on to the other. I've also pulled a wider array of imagery from previous projects. Footballers falling and diving, squirming about in pain on the ground or gymnastically moving through the air, printed from Google searches, ripped from newspapers over many years.

I am drawn in particular to a mass of images I have of the Brazilian footballer Neymar, often seen collapsing, clutching an injured leg, mouth open, hands across his face, arms flailing. His pose, removed from its context, expresses a state of despair, longing and ecstasy, even the suggestion of arousal. The nature of his movements almost balletic, his pose speaking not just of the action on the pitch but now, lifted from it, isolated, conveying an entirely different drama. Occasionally the page will have been ripped to leave the figure reduced to a pair of legs or arms, falling from nowhere. There are books, maps, prints of your poems, textual sources stuck up on the wall and laid across the floor; figures from Titian's *Poesie* paintings enlarged, multiplied, decontextualised; piles of detritus from the burnt-out studio, reminders of different forms of loss and erasure. Slowly these are moved from storage into the studio, readying themselves to become something new.

In the coming weeks I set about trying to obscure and shift this archive, using paint to disrupt the images. I stack them up, letting the puddles of paint soak through the layers, varying in opacity, the fringes of the pools drying to a semi-transparent film, the image ghosting from beneath. Veils of paint are everywhere, the figures and spaces below no longer sitting solidly in optical space but seeming to dissolve. I want to shift the body with these layers of paint, both in image and appearance, moving between solidity and softness, between form and formlessness. The whole, through the layers of paint, becomes reduced to the part, to the fragment, dislocated from its specificity. The body becomes unmoored, able to be entered or occupied by various parties. The single leg, the single hand, the part of a door, the part of a grid or opening. The way these things all start collapsing together within the plane, so that you get both flatness and great depth, a kind of haptic space which is opening and closing at once. Reaching for a mirroring of the vanishing and disappearance of Eurydice at the threshold, for the vanishing I'm witnessing in you. There is a gestation happening, an expansion and serialisation on a theme. The scenes are not episodic, but rather each is a remix and new view, a manic iteration of the same space.

I want these paintings to unbody you, for desire to move beyond the objectified sexual body. I want to spread you across the surface of the canvas, to map the spaces near and far of you, the deep distances of your unknowability and the intimate nature of your love. If Eurydice was scattered in the underworld, then I want each of these studies to be a snapshot of that scattering. I want you to be in continual emergence and disappearance, for these to be surfaces of longing and melancholy. I want to capture the scale of fear around losing you, what that annihilated future might look like, what an obliteration of your presence might feel like.

We are at a Francis Bacon exhibition at the Royal Academy and you stand in a blue dress looking at a triptych from August 1972. It is one of three Bacon made after the suicide of his lover and muse, George Dyer, known collectively as the *Black Triptychs*. You are transfixed. Despite us having walked through room after room of Bacon paintings in this huge exhibition, it is this work which has brought you to a standstill.

Three large canvases in gold frames, each roughly of human proportions, depicting a single figure in a bare room, reduced to geometric forms. A straight line just beneath the halfway point divides a flat grey floor from a beige wall. In the centre of each wall is a doorway, a sharp rectangle of black with a suggestion of a frame to give it the form of an open door. The flanking canvases have triangles of black at the bottom of the floor, tapering in towards the central canvas. They create a border, like the edge of a theatre set. Each depicts the same space, and at the centre of each is a solitary figure in various states of despair. On the left he sits on a chair, right foot raised up to his left knee, the bottom half of the left leg vanishing into the floor. His torso is cut away by the sharp shape of a black shadow, vanishing part of the body into the void of the doorway. His eyes are closed, mouth slightly parted, a three-quarter profile, a smear of white cutting between his mouth and nose. The right panel depicts the same figure, still on the chair, at a moment that could be before or after, the chronology purposefully unclear. His legs are crossed, but the bottom half of them has melted into near-total abstraction. An amorphous pink shape, just clinging to the feel of a leg and a foot, spreads across the floor, or possibly hovers above it, a liquid shadow of flesh. He sits back in the chair, face downturned, head more heavily distorted by scraps and drags of paint, breaking down to the skull beneath. A shadow slices across his torso, creating the feel of a vertical zip opening up the body.

I ask if you remember this triptych from an exhibition of Bacon's work paired with Caravaggio's which we saw in Rome. *Of course.* I rest my hand on the small of your back, feel the soft curve of it with my thumb. You move slowly in front of the three paintings, side to side and back and forth, occasionally sitting on the bench to soak it all in, taking covert snaps of details on your phone.

I remember that exhibition in Rome clearly. In the days leading up to it you were barely able to leave the hotel room, locked to the bed in a sudden pull of depression. I would find you shaking on the bathroom floor, bent over the toilet making yourself sick. When you entered deep sleeps it was hard to know if it was rest for recovery or a further descent. I would leave you sleeping for afternoons to go and seek out various Caravaggio altarpieces, bring you back gifts of jewel-bright jelly sweets and large, sweet oranges in hopes of awakening your hunger for life. In the evenings we would go to small restaurants you had found online. I'd see the way food could bring you such joy, would make you come alive again, the delight of a new flavour or texture. When we first met my diet consisted of bread and nuts, a self-imposed restriction triggered by childhood trauma, but through you I saw the sensuous delight of it, how to turn a fear into joy.

We would spend these nights getting drunk on wine and each other, forgetting the world and remembering our bodies, fucking into feeling something, to feel alive, high on it. In the afternoons when I left you my fears would turn into certainty of finding you dead. I would paint the picture of it in my head before I returned. Each time I found you only asleep, the rise and fall of your chest to each breath a sweet relief. The Bacon and Caravaggio exhibition offered a strange form of hope. You mustered the energy to go, and it surprised me that this exhibition full of violence had been the thing to effect change. Yet that Bacon triptych, for all its despair, seemed to fill you with lightness, connecting you to something which made you feel alive, reconnected to the world, at least temporarily. Paintings as jolts of electricity, life support machines. Perhaps you saw yourself in those works, a language for and recognition of the inexpressible.

In the *Black Triptychs* Bacon is venturing towards a primal and terminal form of lost memory. He is attempting to picture an event without witnesses. To take your own life is to be both perpetrator and victim. All that's left is the aftermath. Bacon described the triptychs as a form of exorcism, experiences which he needed to expel. As if he is trying to enter the room, the moment, that cannot be reached.

I am watching you lost in the picturing of my greatest fear. You are standing barely a foot from the left canvas to capture some close-ups. The gallery lights have cast a shadow of your body, sharply cut across the floor, up the wall, melting into the shadow cast by the canvas itself. The shadow is a bridge, a pathway into the work. I want to climb into that shadow and into the canvas, to turn back out to face you and watch your eyes. What lies in the depths under the surface?

In October 1971 Bacon travelled to Paris for the most important show of his career, a retrospective at the Grand Palais. He'd been estranged from Dyer for some time, but the trip to Paris represented a chance for reconciliation. Dyer had been emotionally and financially dependent on Bacon, and was said to have made various threats and attempts on his own life. They stayed at the Hôtel des Saints-Pères in two rooms with an adjoining bathroom. Dyer arrived sober but soon found himself feeling isolated, and he spiralled into drink. The day before the exhibition's official opening Bacon left Dyer alone to check on the show. All that is known for certain is that Dyer consumed a large amount of alcohol and barbiturates. Bacon was informed of the death, and adopted a mask of calm to continue with his duties at the exhibition in the coming days. The show included numerous canvases depicting Dyer in various states of distress, an actor in a grand theatre of painterly depictions of human suffering. A theatre which had spilt out of the canvases across the bathroom floor of the hotel room.

*

Similar scenes of suffering filled the canvases at the RA show. The body becomes meat, Bacon a butcher opening it up, exposing the internal workings. Figures barely holding on to themselves, exploded across rooms, stages and beds, the spine acting as a pole around which flesh dances and falls. The body in a centrifugal swirl, turning in on itself, but also in the process of exploding outwards. Here is the myth of Bacon, the presumption that his work is a carnival of horror and violence, a great mirror held up to the godless world of pain and suffering that permeates the twentieth century.

You see something different, something beneath and beyond the noise of violence on the surface: under the crashing waves, something deeper, calmer. Great ocean-wide swells of melancholy. You have this tendency to see through things, to see beyond the spectacle. I remember a similar moment with my own work, where I had felt slightly crushed and misunderstood by the singular mode of address, with everyone focused on the horror, seeing my canvases as sites of abjection. Yet you saw, you felt, something beyond this decorative dread, recognising the mourning, the desire for beauty.

We once visited the meticulously reconstructed version of his studio at the Hugh Lane Gallery in Dublin, presented exactly as it was left after his death. A new canvas, covered in the rough sketch of a composition, forever held in the state of possibilities. It is a scene of seeming chaos, made claustrophobic by the sheer amount of material crammed into every corner, piled across the floors, stacked up the walls, with over seven thousand objects in all. Boxes full of pages ripped from magazines and books, newspaper cuttings, stacks of photographs, books, stacks of empty champagne boxes, paint sprayed across the door and ceiling. Canvases are turned to the wall, some ripped or slashed. It is easy to see more pain within this, certainly there is a litany of medical texts focused on the damaged or diseased body, photojournalistic accounts of mutilated bodies in war, scenes from abattoirs. Yet you use a word that Bacon also happened to use a lot. You say it is full of poignancy.

In the weeks after the visit to the RA show I return to the books and archival sources around his studio, with a sense that this sprawling accumulation of materials might act as a kind of archaeological site from which to understand the Dyer triptych further. Or, not really that at all, in an attempt to reach towards what you were feeling and seeing when you were looking at it. In an attempt, through this process, to reach further into the locked doors of you I could not access. As if, somehow, this would help me navigate a way out of the possibility, the dread, of losing you in similar circumstances.

The Dyer triptych, as with all Bacon's work, emerges from this archive. The array of material is astonishing, but these are more than sources. They are working documents, and the ways in which they are manipulated reveal aspects of Bacon's process but also show how these materials became, in their transformations, studies for the final works. There is something closer to jazz than chaos at play here, an artist gathering this material around him over thirty years, manipulating it and becoming intimately familiar with it. It can appear that the material in the studio has been altered by the chaos of the space, the splatters of paint, the rips, the surfaces damaged and covered in marks from the passage of time. Bacon tells David Sylvester that his *photographs are very damaged by people walking over them and crumpling them and everything else, and this does add other implications to an image.* Yet even though these products might seem arbitrary, he has still set up a system in which he allows this damage to take place. He is using chance consciously. He talks of these sources breeding images, but that he wishes to *renew them.* The process is one of germination, sources not dead material but instigators of new life.

How does the figure at the canvas arrive there, from where does it come? The pose of the body in each of the triptych's panels. The cross-legged figure in the left-hand panel appears to be very closely based on a photograph by John Deakin of Dyer sitting in Bacon's studio. Now, in that same studio, a fragment of this painting appears to have been purposefully torn, removing the head, leaving just the bottom half of the body, the figure ripped into a fragment. The rip fragment is covered in the marks and damage of multiple folds, the cracks and creases of this turn the study into something resembling a shard of a shattered stained-glassed window.

Michael Harrison and Rebecca Daniel note the resemblance between this and another ripped-out image in Bacon's studio, where a drawing by Michelangelo sits next to a photograph of the *Apollo Belvedere*. In a number of Bacon's studies there are multiple fragments of figures joined together with a safety pin, tape or paper clip. Bacon acting like Dr Frankenstein, synthetically, surgically building his figures from multiple bodies. The collaged body, part photographic source, part art-historical source, is a figure of multiple migrations, each section decontextualised to find a new body and a new home. The body, the source, the image broken, ready to be rebuilt in paint.

The figure moves further through the process of painting, through an approach that looks to disrupt, enliven and discover. Paint chucked, scrubbed and smeared across the loosely illustrative armature of a sketch, to disorganise the certainty of the figure. Marks which might appear to hold representational weight are, on closer inspection, composed of irrational marks. It is similar to what Bacon sees in a late Rembrandt self-portrait, where the eyes seem to exist without the need or depth of eye sockets, but appear as a result of *a coagulation of non-representational marks*. The irrational and the illustrative marks are entwined, meaning likeness is captured, but remains slippery and fragile. Bacon's citing of that painting is instructive, as it is one which collects up and records time within the paint itself. It shows the artist looking in two directions, across the great spread of what has been and towards the imminence and permeance of death. In the triptych you are viewing similar black holes appear, but in the body itself. The sockets of the eye, the contours of shadows across the torso, passages of dark-ness within the maelstrom of paint. It is a perpetual birth-death cycle, where the figure moves simultaneously towards oblivion and towards life, form both forming and unforming. As Gilles Deleuze states, *the body attempts to escape from itself through one of its organs in order to rejoin the field or material structure.*

The figure in the central panel of the triptych is perhaps the most alarming manifestation of this movement. Laid horizontal across the floor, half the body splayed across the entrance to the dark, the other half spilling like liquid into the room, the cer-tainty of the form as figure dissolving. The head is abandoned of features, an empty death mask, a scrubbed-up set of absences, a shape only just holding on to the appearance of a head, the jut of a chin, a shadow which seems to blindfold the eyes and the curve of the forehead clinging on to eligibility. It is mainly con-text that lets us read these vague forms as the left-over shapes of a vanished face attached to the sack-like form of a body. It is caught in a devastating trap, the gymnastics of the figure a final spasm from life into death. The painting and the body as sites for these grand theatrics, for this existential magician's trick. A vanishing.

A pink circular form, neither quite blood nor shadow, spills out of the body and across the floor. The pink pool is the body shifting from flesh to spirit, from presence to absence. It is falling, not downwards, but rather working as if against gravity, flesh breaking away, siphoned out of the body, filtered towards nothingness. The contours of the body are softer, no longer the violent deformation of line we see in the other bodies but the contour as permeable barrier, what Deleuze calls *a curtain where the Figure shades off into infinity*. The figure is not being seen through this curtain, this curtain is part of a body in the process of moving through its own borders to join the gap between figure and structure. This thin film is the space through which and into which the figure is falling into what Deleuze accurately calls a *cosmic dissipation, in a closed but unlimited cosmos*. The nature of the fall, in spatial and temporal terms, is both infinitesimal and infinite.

Bacon was a keen reader of Shakespeare, and the neurosis of the paintings seems closer to Hamlet's worrying than anything else. They are a staging of Hamlet's *O that this too too solid flesh would melt,/Thaw, and resolve itself into a dew*. Those scrubs and that pink pool oozing from Dyer's body are the residue, are the melted flesh, the resolution of the body into dew.

To become and unbecome. Spirit and flesh. It is exactly what I am trying to paint of you, but spread out across the entire canvas. I found myself returning to the Hugh Lane Gallery, to Bacon's studio and the chaotic-seeming archive, as if I might find clues there about how to paint you, about how to get at the vanishing that was taking place in front of me. If, somehow, I might take that archive as a starting point from which to build a new body of paintings.

Bacon owned a copy of *Phenomena of Materialisation*, an early-twentieth-century book by Baron von Schrenck-Notzing, a German physician, psychiatrist and researcher of psychic phenomenon. The book is well worn, with various pages ripped out, folded and covered in painty fingerprints. Michael Harrison and Rebecca Daniels cite various examples where these images acted as sources for Bacon's paintings across his career. The book records a number of theatrical and contentious seances which von Schrenck-Notzing documented and researched, believing the spirits conjured to be genuine. They centre on a French medium called Eva Carrière and demonstrate her ability to conjure ectoplasm and the appearance of lives from another realm. The mainly male audience at the performances were said to have had sexual acts performed on them, and to have been witnesses to Eva's partner inserting two fingers into her vagina to check for ectoplasm. It is thought that such erotic theatrics made them more pliable, all cynicism exiting through the phallic blindness of their gaze, the blinkered vision of sexual desire. The same could be said of Bacon, the virtuosity of his paint a form of arousal which allows us, even temporarily, to leave all cynicism at the door, to believe momentarily that the spirit of Dyer is here, crossing the curtained divide of the painting, reaching out to touch. It points back to the Dyer triptych, towards the idea of Bacon not as just the painter of fleshy violence but also of ghosts.

Perhaps the making of unseen forces of transience seen was his preoccupation? In many of his paintings he depicts grass, seemingly sprouting from nowhere, whisking in the wind. They all seem to source the same photograph. Bacon mentions the photograph and its transformation to Sylvester, saying *it was a marvellous photograph I have of grass, and the photograph had got torn up and it formed to some extent the shape that the grass has. It kept on being trampled on so much in all the chaos of where I work, and, when I pulled it out, it had practically all fallen away, but there was just this sort of fragment of grass left.* It is this process of the image being trampled into submission, of it having *practically fallen away.* There is a duality to the crumbled and trampled photograph, the image of the wind in grass and the state of the image as fading back into the surface through the pressures and marking of many feet. In both cases the passing of time are recorded, the hidden forces of time, be that the wind which only shows itself through effect, or passing pressures of feet, which render not their presence but record themselves through the vanishing of the image. Both the wind and the feet, unseen, render visible memory and time itself, both passing as ghosts through the image. It is a desire to hold on to transience itself.

This desire shows itself in his use of dust in his paintings, gathered from the studio floor. He comments to Sylvester that *dust seems to be eternal – seems to be the one thing that lasts forever,* and later suggests he is unsure how stable it is in terms of conservation, musing that he does not *know about the lastingness of things.* Yet the phrase seems to speak more broadly, to this sense of sadness at the impermanence of everything, which dust seems, paradoxically, to capture. The dust in his studio is of course made up of cells shed from the skin, the hair, the fibrous detritus of clothes and the slow rain of all objects undressing themselves across time. Looking at dust under a microscope is like looking into the dark of space, a night sky scarred with pinholes, dashes and fragments of light, shards of what was life now turned into a microscopic intergalactic landscape. Zoom in closer and the fragments become comets, whole planets floating in space. There is beauty to the way things seem to sparkle and crystallise here, the patterning of dead matter now a glittering constellation. When our skin is sloughed off we are casting whole microscopic galaxies into the world. That Bacon should gather handfuls of this dead matter and use it in his paintings to render new life is him flinging stardust into paint.

One of the constants of Bacon's studio is his circular mirror, a legacy to his time as an interior designer. The surface of the mirror is a moon, distressed and milky, damaged by time. A moon working its singular gravity on the studio, on the artist, pulling him in, controlling the rhythm of the tides. It is no longer a surface that can possibly offer up a sharp reflection, but rather one that will distort the world. Deleuze comments that for Bacon, in his paintings, mirrors are many things, but never reflective surfaces, he says *nothing is behind the mirror, everything is inside it.* I think this runs further than the mirrors Bacon depicts in his paintings. This is exactly what his paintings do. They don't reflect the world, they are the other side of the mirror. Bacon references Cocteau when discussing death, who said, *each day in the mirror I watch death at work.* Cocteau's Orpheus enters the underworld through a mirror, and similar motifs appear throughout his work. Martin Harrison believes that a still from Cocteau's film *Le Sang d'un poète* (*The Blood of a Poet*) (1932) might have had a direct influence on Bacon's painting *Jet of Water* (1979). In the still a figure can be seen leaping from the floor into a frame, which could be a mirror, a window, an opening or even a painting. As the figure crosses into the surface and into the space beyond, waves of water splash back outwards. The image seems more than just a possible reference point for Bacon's imagery, it is an encapsulation of what his Dyer triptychs do; they similarly encounter this two-way movement, into the mirror, into the painting, into the underworld. If Cocteau is one of the great retellers of Orpheus' entrance into the underworld, into death, in the quest to find his love, it is possible that Bacon is another. But his retelling escapes narrative, holds us in a constant cycle at this key point of expansion and contraction, at the threshold, at the entrance and exit point, a culmination of all the drama at the border, all of it circling around the membrane between us and death.

This is where Bacon is, where we are, in front of those Dyer paintings. We are Orpheus, Dyer is Eurydice, the surface of the painting as the threshold between realms. Even in the godless atheism of Bacon the underworld exists. Even when it is the space of our grief, our love, where the other goes and where they haunt us from. What could be more tragic than a quest in which there is not the possibility of the questing narrative, in which we are held forever in the spinning cataclysm of the borderspace, only able to look in. The lover's quest for the lost, the dead, the other who is in oblivion, truly annihilated, the lover who searches in a void, aware of the paradox, aware of the utter impossibility of the search, but is still pulled in by the magnitude and gravity of grief. What might we see there, what might that underworld contain? Is it really, truly nothing, or is it hungry, devouring everything?

Bacon's life was shot through with death, from that of his brother to those of a multitude of friends and lovers. He once commented that *people have been dying around me like flies*. Considering the Dyer paintings and Bacon's biography, loaded with loss after loss, I wonder if, like Keats, his great subject is not so much death as grief, and therefore love. Grief is the mirror image of love, the consequence of companionship, desire and connection. Grief can be as unending and vast as the forever-expanding universe. Grief can be the architect of an entire underworld.

Watching you look at the Dyer triptych, it strikes me that all of this entire underworld is here. It's a great spectral swirl, gathering like clouds of invisible dust between you and the canvas. Not just the grief, but the library of books, the studio full of studies, the interviews, the love, the pain, the entire network. Perhaps this is Bacon's accidental offering up of an atheist underworld. Not one that can be entered, or believes in an afterlife of a spirit or a soul. Rather an underworld which resides in that split moment, in the gap and membrane that exist in painting and the body at the moment of death. That space, between you and the painting, between the end and grieving, the distance of lost lovers.

I consider how to solidify what I am painting and how I might paint you or the underworld. I feel haunted by images, they seem to keep coming to me even when I don't want them to, and I am not able to escape the tangents of associations. They are not taking me closer to a form of picturing you, and in this spiral they are taking me further away. Lines from Deleuze on Bacon catch my attention. *Suppose the Figure had effectively disappeared, leaving behind only a vague trace of its former presence. The field will then open up like a vertical sky.* I had been pushing towards the wiped zones of his paintings and the sites of disappearance. I wished to paint the trace alone, the wide-open space of *a vertical sky.* Perhaps I needed to focus on emergence, a form of abstraction which might contain unbodied life.

I manage to get hold of a number of the texts that Bacon had in his studio, including the *Phenomena of Materialisation: A Contribution to the Investigation of Mediumistic Teleplastics* by Baron von Schrenck-Notzing. The contemporaneous sensationalised responses to the case focus largely on the erotic nature of the encounters, whereas the diary and accompanying photographs of the seances reveal a more complex picture. I'm more interested in what von Schrenck-Notzing believes he saw than what was real or possible.

Eva is treated like a medical specimen. Her skull is measured, teeth counted, the entire body mapped in meticulous and invasive detail. He considers her *undisturbed.* For him, *her special faculty consists entirely in the production of materially formed bodies, beginning in barely visible and optically cloud-like or amor-phous structures, and ending in the formation of solid materials, or organic shapes.*

His records include diagrams of the set-up of rooms for each seance. This involved an assortment of chairs for an audience, a flashlight camera positioned to capture the appearances and a curtained-off area where Eva would be stationed in a trance-like state triggered by hypnosis. The photographs often show Eva behind the curtain, sitting in the dark, eyes closed, with her two hands holding the opening of the fabric. Often other hands, normally appearing from outside the frame, appear holding on to Eva's. One tends to be male and one female. The curtains are then closed, and all that can be seen is the hands crossing and holding each other. Then, white mists gather into molten liquids, and long, fleshy forms like umbilical cords sprout from Eva's body, falling into the hands of the witness figures. Faces, hands and bodies, at first ghostly, appear from the dark, or from her body, then step free, shifting from spirit to flesh. An ejaculatory form flows from her mouth like a huge wave, then takes the shape of an arm, a hand sprouting from its end. Hands like inverted shadows, malleable forms reaching, touching and covering the body. In other photographs her face, her entire body, seems to vanish and all that is left are the emergent forms. Growths emerge from her neck, as if second heads wearing dis-torted masked faces. These heads grow into deformed organic shapes and then detach, floating from the body of the host. Eva's face shifts from its expressionless detachment to contracted con-tortions of pain. A menacing male face spreads across a floating lump of flesh and stares back out at us. Later Eva seems to be accompanied by her double, in a face resembling a death mask. Life emerges from darkness. Bodies born from nothingness, arriving from another realm.

Police are sent to Eva's apartment to find proof of fraud. Convincing evidence is provided to suggest that the fleshy forms are chewed-up paper and the faces are merely manipulated copies of newspaper cuttings, including an altered photograph of President Woodrow Wilson. Is the whole thing absurd, even comical, a cheap magician's trick? The diaries suggest that all involved believed in the supernatural appearances. Perhaps Baron von Schrenck-Notzing was seeing what he wanted to see or was an accomplice in the delusion. Perhaps Eva and Juliette were cheap con artists. But are we not still haunted, even if someone can prove that the ghosts did not exist?

What of the flashlight photos? Are they records of events that happened, or does the camera conjure the ghosts? Photography is a form which does not just distil and represent reality but which constructs its own. Could my studio too be a theatre, paint a medium to conjure ghosts? In painting the curtained-off space of Eva's seance, I can see what forms might meet me.

In the back of my studio is a box of stuff we have collected through our various pregnancies, including packs of polaroid film. We intended to record your body's changes, and then our children, our child, in the first days and weeks after birth. Something about the physical immediacy of the polaroid, the fact you couldn't take endless snaps, appealed to us. We never had the chance to use them, and now they read as images and moments that would never exist.

Polaroid film holds all the chemical ingredients for both the capturing and processing of the photographic image. The film is the site of its own development. It contains both the positive and negative layer of a photograph, and little pockets of emulsion and chemicals are stored at the base of the camera. These are released when the photograph is taken, the mixture of chemicals and layers determining how the light is captured, translated and fixed on the sheet. All of this becomes visible when the film leaves the camera. The image slowly appears, like one of the ghosts conjured by Eva.

I imagine reversing the process to conjure you. Ripping open the sealed boxed of polaroid film, I bring them into the light. The colour sheets turn immediately brown, the black and white ones grey, two flat sheets acting like primed surfaces. I squeeze out the chemicals from the little pockets at the bottom, at first between my thumb and forefinger and then using the edge of a debit card to reach every last drop. The ink comes out in bulging bubbles of blue, pushing up from inside at the taut surface of the polaroid film. There are twenty-four sheets in total, and slowly I figure out what the chemicals do, how I can work them up and across the surface from within the layers. I manipulate them with my fingers, with the debit card, turning it on its edge to draw the chemicals in a line. Over time the chemicals reveal different tones and colours. If gently bent, the liquids crack and split across the surface, so that a small pocket of air temporarily opens between the internal layers. The liquids create forms, surfaces and the suggestion of space. As I work on them one by one they inform each other, each one suggesting possibilities for the next.

A number of them take the shape of natural forms, a geode or geological cross section of strata. Slices of agate, a vast mountain range, a wide expanse of ice, cracking and breaking, in the process of melting. The white foam of the sea's surf. The edge of land, the tide sweeping up across its expanse, snowfall, an avalanche, the deepest corners of an ocean, a sky falling in. An opening, perhaps into a cave. A frozen forest, a subterranean pool of water. Some are more nebulous, the vague suggestion of being submerged, or caught shifting between states, a slow unfurling from solid through liquid and into gas. Things rise, fall, appear and disappear. At points the imagery looks purely aerial, seeds scattered high and wide in the sky.

Elsewhere, bodies. Often opened up, without clarity of form, contours dissolved, pure liquid spilling. Microscopic views of matter, the enlarged world of some kind of living organism. Landscapes of blood, cellular structures, systems of life support, embryonic matter, foetal forms. A curtain. A veil. Pure light endlessly spreading out, reaching towards us and into the deep distance. These are images arriving from nothing, not the world captured as was intended but formed from the chemical matter. I see you everywhere in these psychological hinterlands, your internal world made visible. Here are the landscapes of the underworld, wandered endlessly. Spaces at the edge of a world, at the slipping points between. I want to find you here.

In a letter to John Baur, the American painter Joan Mitchell wrote, *I paint from remembered landscapes that I carry with me – and remembered feelings of them, which of course become transformed. I could certainly never mirror nature. I would like more to paint what it leaves me with.* I carry the landscapes of you with me. I know I cannot fully enter the hidden underworld of your psyche, but I want to paint what it leaves me with. These are landscapes of feelings, transformed by the transference of our exchange and memories.

The possibility of a baby started to feel remote. Each test seemed to erase another path. We were now alone in a barren landscape, with a thick, transparent layer of glass between us, all sound muffled. To look up was to see the vertical sky viewed through the ceiling of a deep ocean, light fading.

Slowly time stitches things back together. The landscape populated with new paths, the ceiling of the ocean peeling back, water flooding upwards to paint the sky. We breathe again.

Various experimental medical options reveal themselves. Our specialist suggests another endometrial scratch as it might make the lining of your womb *fussier*, meaning it less likely for unviable embryos to be taken on. She prescribes you progesterone, to help in the early stages of pregnancy. The final option is an experimental drug which they think might make the womb less prone to taking on unviable embryos. We sign up to the trial.

Our friends Daisy and Matt had their first baby a few weeks after the twins were due. Shortly after his first birthday they send us a cryptic text saying they need to talk, and I am a hive of anxiety, certain that it must be some kind of intervention to address how we have not been great friends over the last year or two. I am flooded with guilt. They want to meet in person, so we wait nervously for them at our house. The air seems thicker, everything compressing inwards. They tell us that they are planning to try for a second child soon, and wanted us to know. That they are trying now because after having a second they would like to offer, should we still be struggling, the option of Daisy being a surrogate. I look at you and for a moment or two your face is totally blank. Then I see it sink in incrementally, and there is a beauty to the way your face, your body, your eyes now lock on to mine and seem to mirror exactly what I am feeling. We are both flooded with love, overwhelmed by it. For the rest of their stay I feel outside my body, dislocated from the world, can't quite digest or process the scale and beauty of the offer or that two friends should even think to suggest this. The magnitude of their love dazzles and dazes me. I'm unable to articulate how grateful I am.

In the coming days we are knocked mute by it, then become lifted into loquaciousness. It feels as if we have been gifted another path and reminded of the astonishing circles of love that surround us. The loneliness we had been feeling was a mirage.

We are slowly coming out of a deep sleep, and in our awakening we see a surround of faces, of friends and family.

Strangely, the sense of new paths allows us to settle into the other possibility that we may, through circumstances or eventually choice, end up without a child. We had been frozen by the fear of this. Yet now it seems as if a child is a want rather than a need, something we desire but are able to contemplate not having. It feels liberating that this might be a path we come to actively choose. As a result, bit by bit I can feel you coming back. The fear of losing you is slipping away, as if the choices have liberated us from what seemed like a headlong plummet towards annihilation. We are finding pleasure in the world, in the small things, in each other. We are escaping from living in the permanent future, settling back into the heat and aliveness of the now.

In the studio I have started to draw you again. You are all edge. The lie of the drawn figure, of the two-dimensional version, the edge a containable thing. The body, the figure, the image as a thing that cannot map, not truly, the other. The coordinates and borders, the flattened image that can be circum-navigated. Whatever their complexity, drawings are merely the bordered edge of an island's map. But I am exploring the island. The edge, the edges of you. The edges of a lover. The edge is continuous. The edge as the skin of the body, the edge as that space the eye, the finger, the tongue might explore. Sight and touch inextricably linked in the eroticism of desire. To look is to desire and think through touch, to touch is to see anew. To trace, to map, to see afresh and to know, or get closer to knowing. The reciprocal movement, touch as unspoken dialogue, constant tiny movements in pressure, in placement. Each touch a question, or a questioning, each movement a recognition, a mode of permission. A conversation. Each movement across each other a slow opening up of the self, of the body. A letting in.

8

Scatter

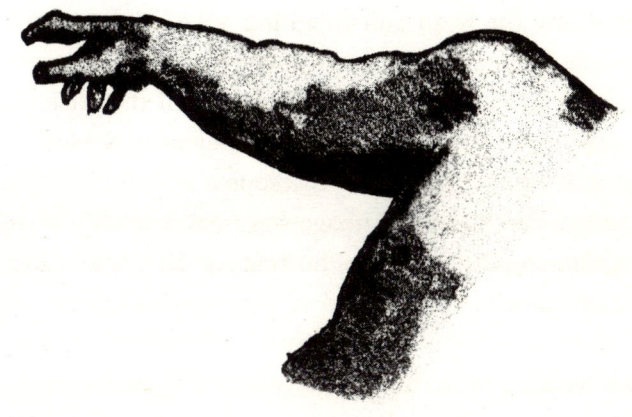

We see what we want to see. In 1988 Gerhard Richter completed his cycle of fifteen paintings known as *October 18, 1977*. On that date, Jan-Carl Raspe, Andreas Baader and Gudrun Ensslin are found dead in their prison cells. They were senior members of the Baader-Meinhof group, an underground anti-establishment collective, active in West Germany from the early 1970s. They were left-wing extremists, using violence and terror to fund their attempts to overturn what they saw as the oppression of the state. Richter said, *The deaths of the terrorists, and the related events both before and after, stand for a horror that distressed me and has haunted me as unfinished business ever since, despite all my efforts to suppress it.* His paintings appear like efforts to exorcise these ghosts, or at least to picture the haunting.

Three of the paintings are based on a photograph of Ulrike Meinhof after her death published in *Stern* magazine on 16 June 1976. The pose is reminiscent of Hans Holbein's *The Body of the Dead Christ in the Tomb* (*c*.1520–22), one of the most iconic German paintings of the dead Christ in history. In Richter's painting only the head and shoulders are seen in profile, the suggestion of the eyes open, the mouth parted in release of a final breath upwards, into the deep black of the background. Across the three versions the head is increasingly blurred in a staged shift from reality, from the source and from life. In the final canvas the body and image have become soft, diffused, shifting from solidity. They are portraits of the brutal, mournful, permanent isolation of death.

Another painting is from a police photograph of Gudrun Ensslin hanging in her cell. The image is framed by a murky, curtain-like form which almost becomes pure shadow. It enacts death. Behind the figure is a gridded window, the boundary between the two threatened by the blurring of the contours, meaning the figure and the space, the foreground and the background, are dissolving into each other. Her legs are nearly totally vanished into streaks of light, giving the impression of the body floating in space. The body, the room and the image are turning into ghostly apparitions. They are the hauntings a distressed Richter had tried to suppress, finally given form.

Andreas Baader's empty cell is depicted in another painting, the vertical lines of the room and the bookshelves drags of dramatic downward movement, towards a floor vanished entirely, leaving a space of total darkness. The static nature of the source image has been transformed into a scene of total motion, the permanent stasis of death given a dramatic form of movement, as if capturing the process of shifting from life into death.

Richter blurs the paint by moving still-wet paint across the flat surface of the canvas. The dried surfaces retain a memory of previous liquidity. Where the drag marks are more pronounced the paint will have been already drying, in the process of stitching itself back together. The painting shifts from liquid into solid while the image shifts from solidity into liquidity: moving in opposing directions. We are in the hinterland of ambiguity and transience.

Terry Mullen first heard of the Baader-Meinhof Group in 1994, then days later saw another mention of them in an article. He was startled enough by the coincidence to write a letter to a newspaper, sparking a small flurry of responses from readers who cited similar incidences. It would become known colloquially as the Baader-Meinhof phenomenon, before later being coined as the frequency illusion by a linguistics professor, Arnold Zwicky, in 2005. Zwicky suggested that the frequency illusion was the meeting of selective attention bias and confirmation bias, meaning the effect is caused by our ability to see only what we deem to be important, filtering out the vast sum of other noise and drawing information which supports our thesis. Sight becomes not an objective engagement with reality but a deconstruction and reconstruction of the reality we want to perceive.

I'm haunted by these kinds of illusions. I wonder if all the paintings I have been making really are full of the things I thought I felt and saw in them, or if the connections I am seeing are products of my imagination. What if my paintings, and everything else, are apparitions, projections, mere sites of desire. I am certainly seeing death everywhere, the losses triggering a kind of hyper-frequency illusion.

After the tests, the trials, the medication, the scratch, the waiting and the exploration of alternatives, you are pregnant again. Yet even in that thin pink line confirming the start and possibility of life, I see the inevitability of death. I think we both do, the excitement of early tests replaced not even with the crippling anxiety of the last few, but a kind of dull ache of certainty that this will be temporary. It might even be fair to say we are bored.

You start cramping after a fortnight, and we know what to associate that with now, but blood doesn't come. We book a scan, sure of the outcome. The day of the appointment, one of our cats brings in a blackbird egg, green-blue and cracked. She must have held it delicately in her mouth for it to survive the journey inside, then dropping it on the carpet to allow the shell to split into spiders' webs. Both our cats are useless hunters so such occurrences are rare, but I wasn't surprised. We had seen an excessive amount of roadkill on the way to hospital visits and doctor's appointments. Badgers, squirrels, a muntjac. Returning from the last meeting with our consultant, a fox and her cub caught either side of the central reservation of the motorway. This disturbed us deeply.

We convince ourselves that the things we are seeing in the world are a confirmation of our internal psyche. We paint our own poetic fallacies through what we subconsciously notice. I'd spent the previous evening drawing blackbirds for a special edition of David Almond's iconic novel *Skellig*. Skellig is a man with wings, a figure lifted from the world of William Blake and dumped in the derelict garage at the bottom of a family garden. After all these drawings of blackbirds, here was a cracked egg lying on the floor of my home, stolen from the nest, a safe space neatly split open and spilt across the floor. I felt a little broken by the sight, by the delicacy of the eggshell, by the loss. By the omen of it. I lifted it carefully on to a piece of tissue and put it by the side of my desk.

The cramping is worse, so we are resigned as you lie back on the padded gurney. No tears in your eyes, only a glassy stare elsewhere. I hold your hand, squeeze as the probe goes in, rotates, searches. On screen, a cone-shaped void of white noise, glimmering pulses of light against dark. Nothing. They continue looking, concerned the nothing could indicate another ectopic pregnancy. Then slowly, at the centre, coming into soft focus, a little dark circle. We squint our eyes, watch it take firmer shape. *That's the gestational sac.* My heart throbs. Your face is still carefully poised. *I'm just looking for signs of the foetal pole and yolk sac.* I squint, not understanding her words, but willing there to be a sign of something inside the black hole, but nothing. She points out the *bright endometrial reaction*, a soft white line, a thin glowing border. They take careful measurements. They measure again, and again, and double-check the measurements against a chart. *I'm afraid that it is measuring closer to five weeks than six.* You stare into nothingness. *I don't want you to give up hope, but there is a chance growth might have stopped at five weeks.* They ask us to return in a week, when they are hoping to see signs of a foetal pole.

The drive home is silent. I keep glancing over at you, your face a mask. I'm not sure where you are. I didn't see any dead animals on the way home, I am not sure I see anything at all.

For a week everything seems to freeze.

I google foetal pole and the description comes up as *the thickening on the margin of the yolk sac of a foetus during pregnancy.* On the margin, that feels like where we now are, waiting. You keep the printout of the scan by the bed. We do the normal round of telling people the situation, while not really knowing. Each morning and each night I hold the print in my hands, will the little pole into being. Perhaps what we have seen in this blurred image is not total stasis, but merely delayed movement forwards. Perhaps our dates are wrong. At night when we hold each other I think into that dark space. Swim little fish, swim. Your fear is palpable, amplified through the house, through your body. But I hold on to it, because it means you are hoping, too.

Yet hope is slowly taken over by the visions of death. It imprints itself on to everything. Even in this evidence of growth, of the possibility of early development, all I can see is loss. The shadowing of the past deaths and a foreshadowing of what feels like the inevitability of more in the future. The black hole not as a space for that pole to live and grow in, but one which reads to me like a microscopic coffin. You are wandering the vast, cavernous space of this tiny coffin inside you.

A week later we return for the follow-up scan. The white noise again, and for a long while nothing, then the black circle, where we hope to have seen growth, where we would expect a life forming inside, but nothing, no yolk sack or foetal pole. Nothing. She keeps looking, scanning, the gestational sac shifting in and out of focus. We convince ourselves that there is a flicker of something in the shadows. Surely we can't see anything, are just willing it to be ... then slowly it comes into view, increases sharpness, and there it is, shimmering in and out of sight, a white, nebulous shape. *Yes.*

Yes?

Yes. That is the foetal pole, which is exactly what we would want to be seeing, and there is the yolk sac. Then a tiny flickering.

Is that?

Yes. It starts with a little flutter. A heartbeat.

How to paint into this? The polaroid paintings suggested a different path, that it might be possible to work towards forms,

148

spaces, images and modes of life which were not preconceived or designed, but which were led by and emerging from the process. Painting as a form of self-creation, a self-sustaining mode of world-building. This work had felt like a hopeful act, a way to construct models of space and life that were determined by the internal logic of the paintings. The photographic canvases were openings into an underworld which formed itself step by step, which saw itself expand layer by layer. The polaroids suggested the possibility that landscape, architecture and the body need not be separate entities within the space of a painting, but that they could coalesce. That the presumed boundaries and certainties which normally separate these entities could dissolve. Perhaps the underworld could be this type of space, a new architecture. Perhaps the space in which I find you, and picture you, might be here. In one of your Eurydice poems she wonders, *How will I tempt another summer to/seek me here, in this well/of embalming dark.* The painting is this light in the *embalming dark*, seeking you in the recesses of an underworld. Painting is a mode of embalming, of holding and pausing the darkness. Might I paint to *tempt another summer*, arriving suddenly with that heartbeat?

I unfold the large stack of painted, unstretched canvases which had been stacked up in piles in the studio. Our house is being renovated, and I've collected the stripped-out parts of the house to use as material. Floorboards riddled with woodworm dragged into the studio, window panes and frames and a set of rusted steel beams. I pile them up next to the various burnt objects from the fire, paint pots, book covers, stretcher bars, charred rectangular boards, a door. I have stacks of metal grids of different size and thickness, offcuts of things used by the builders, others collected from the local rubbish tip. I've moss and branches from the forest and along the river, branches. From the garden I've kept weeds, detritus and sliced the trunk of a dead, felled horse chestnut tree into cross sections to use.

These objects will guide the paint, lay out the composition, act as stencils. On one of the canvases I lay down the floorboards in roughly organised vertical strips, making a series of diagonals. Mixing up a thick, syrupy paint, I pour it into a spray gun, cover the entire canvas to create a thin sheen of semi-translucent dark crimson across the surface. Days later I will remove the boards, feel them sticky where the paint grips the edges. Beneath them the negative space, the arteries of colour and layers not covered by the crimson curtain. I repeat the process across various canvases, and on some the layering continues, the colour, the nature of the mixture and the tone changing. In the more successful surfaces are the sense of a house seen through an X-ray, or a building collapsing, the floor rising up to become a wall, an opened-up ceiling, a detonation of space. It's not clear that these surfaces are constructed from the spaces left by the floorboards, but there is a nod and echo to domestic interiors, a room opened out in surprising ways, a stage collapsed under its own weight. When I hang the loose canvases up vertically the effect is discombobulating, the surfaces so clearly referencing floors, but ones lifted upwards, the interior of a house gathered into a Wizard of Oz-style tornado, thrown across an unknown sky. The underworld now a series of rooms where we can walk, not just across but in vertical lines, ascending and descending as if in one of Escher's Penrose Triangle illusions.

Marks are indexical signs which quickly become divorced from what they signify. The shape left by a book might carry no memory or suggestion of the book, but will become many other things. The objects themselves, in return, are changed. They gather paint, they get covered in the memories of the process. They are no longer merely tools but become sculptural paintings, collecting up the stains and accidents of the paintings' histories. The paint abstracts the objects, but also sets up a dialogue with them. There is no hierarchy, a polyphonic set of interrelations. The paint-covered objects are holders of memories, but ones we might not be able to access. History recorded that eludes the viewer.

The organic materials gathered from the garden, and from forest and river walks have a different effect. I scatter them across surfaces, spray thin mists of paint across them to capture the subtle specificity of their shapes. The stencils retain outlines of lavender, a branch, a rose, a leaf, a clutch of wild grass or the tiny cut-out shapes of a daisy. These negative shapes are direct memories and indexes which hold firm to the root. They create surfaces like the reflections and refractions which tumble across a river, with uncertain depths and liquid confusion. When these shadows interact with the architectural spaces it is as if everything is being seen through the surface of a river. I see a musical dissolving of inside and outside, rooms filled to the brim with rivers flowing upwards. How might an underworld be built, and what place might we construct for a lover in its depths?

A photograph of the lover. The photo, by Jasper Johns, appears to be taken from a seated position, mirroring its primary subject, the artist Robert Rauschenberg. He sits crossed-legged on a low-lying wooden table, laden with a mirror, a stack of documents, a mug and a vase of flowers. The latter are casting smudged layers of shadow across the wood-panelled walls. The flowers appear to be carnations, a symbol of love. It is unlikely that the photograph was intended to be seen by a wide public. So the viewer, in stepping into Johns' place, is entering an intimate and private encounter of one lover observing the other.

Rauschenberg and Johns were in the middle of an intense

six-year creative and romantic partnership. They never publicly declared themselves as lovers, so there were contentions around the literature outing them. Rauschenberg married Susan Weil in 1950, but they separated two years later, having had one child. Rauschenberg's romantic relationship with the artist Cy Twombly was sandwiched between his marriage and the relationship with Johns.

Next to Rauschenberg, just beneath him on the floor, are a scattered array of pens and pencils and an industrial-sized bottle of lighter fluid. His left hand holds a piece of paper while masking the site of his right hand and the motions and marks it is making on to the unseen plane. It is 1958 and they are in their Front Street studio in New York, Rauschenberg working on one of the thirty-six drawings he would make to illustrate cantos from Dante's *Inferno*.

A few years ago we went to see a retrospective of Rauschenberg's work in London. It was a huge, sprawling show and we ended up walking around at different speeds. When we returned home we found we'd bought each other a postcard of the same work: *Canto XIV: Circle Seven, Round 3, The Violent Against God, Nature, and Art* (1960). We both still have the postcard on our writing desks, little cardboard mirrors in which we had seen something of the other. What was it we saw there? Where were we when we both seemed to find the other?

The *Inferno* is the first of three parts in Dante's epic poem the *Divine Comedy*, written between 1308 and 1321. The poem sees Dante enter the gates of Hell, guided by the Roman poet Virgil, where they journey through the underworld to confront the suffering of sinners. The poem organises Hell into nine concentric circles, each descending spatially to correspond with a hierarchy of sin, with Satan awaiting at the central and deepest point. The punishments of the sinners are set up in relation to their sin, a moral rhyme of poetic justice. Each circle is subdivided in the poem by a series of cantos, the structuring of the text acting as an allegorical architecture.

Rauschenberg's reimaginings are small works on paper, each made up of a series of transferred images with layered additions of pen and paint. Each artwork, like each stanza and canto of the poem, acts like a portal, leading us further into the depths of Hell. They are spaces that invite us in, as joint explorers. Virgil leads Dante, as Dante leads the reader, as Rauschenberg leads us. We are led, canto by canto, page by page, into the descending *depthless-deep*:

> *Death-pale, the Poet spoke:*
> *Now let us go*
> *Into the blind world waiting here below us.*

Eventually, we arrive at the seventh circle (*Canto XIV: Circle Seven, Round 3, The Violent Against God, Nature, and Art*), sunk deep in Hell now, reaching the sins deemed the most egregious. A vast horizonless desert, sand burning under our feet, all growth, all hope burnt away. Rain descends as fire. Supposed sinners cast to the depths of Hell for the crime of sodomy. The price of love in the hands of Christian dogma, where bodily and spiritual autonomy is eradicated in the face of divine judgement.

The page is split into two sections by a horizontal line, three-quarters of the way up the page. At the centre of this top strip is a red-chalk outline of a right foot, presumed to be the artist's own. It is a starkly different form of drawing and bodily representation to anything else in the series, in its outlining of an actual body part. The edges of the foot are soft. The chalk has been rubbed into a warm pink, creating the semi-solidity of flesh. To the left, a series of comparatively tiny footprints have been laid into the paper via the transfer technique. If the footsteps are a crossing of the border, an entrance into the burning plain, then the large red foot is resolutely stood at the threshold. We are able to imaginatively step into the space left by the foot, for our foot to be housed in the outline around Rauschenberg's. The space of the I becomes shared. The collective I looks down into the seventh circle.

What we see is a teeming mass of characters, in various states of dissolution, arriving here via literal transference. Rauschenberg uses materials and imagery sourced from mass media as the basis for his illustrations. A print laid face down on to the sheet of paper, the back of the paper coated with lighter fluid. The liquid would seep through the layers, loosening the ink from the paper, creating a layer of liquidity between the two sheets. He would then apply pressure with a pencil or pen, transferring the ink from one skin to another, exchanging the fluids between two surfaces.

Rauschenberg's Dante drawings arrive at the point when Abstract Expressionism was the dominant language in American art. There could barely be a starker dismissal of the ideals of Abstract Expressionism than to illustrate an Italian Renaissance poem, using the materials and imagery of everyday life. Rauschenberg was consciously entering into a rich history of such responses to Dante's poem by Sandro Botticelli, Gustave Doré and William Blake. Rauschenberg's approach was to capture the entirety of a canto within the limits of each drawing's individual frame, creating a direct correspondence between the space of a drawing and the space of the poetic canto.

It's a poem written in a world where believers had potent hallucinogenic visions of such hellscapes. Rauschenberg's approach filtered the poem through the language, materials and conditions of the present moment to capture the spirit of Dante, building an underworld from the ephemeral materiality of the present. Mass media was the vehicle through which the mythology of mid-twentieth-century America was built, so it made perfect sense to build a lexicon around its discarded fragments. The ephemera of the everyday is lifted to construct the eternal depths of the afterlife, to transport the poem from fourteenth-century Italy to mid-twentieth-century America. From the detritus of one world he builds an underworld which we are not just moved through, but which we are invited to explore.

It means that the figures in all the *Inferno* works are bodies in exile, departed from one world and entering another. Hell becomes the perfect location for such a dislocation, souls lifted from the detritus of the everyday and entered into new eternal states of damnation and classification. It is part of a continued filtering which runs through Rauschenberg's entire oeuvre.

Surprisingly, Titian's *Poesie* paintings offer a way in. In an earlier work, *Small Rebus* (1956), Rauschenberg incorporated a photograph of Titian's *The Rape of Europa*. The print of the painting is black and white and has been cut down on both sides. It is positioned at the bottom-left edge of the artwork, giving the impression that the image is entering from outside the frame. To the right of the print is a white rectangle of paint, with a few lines at the top, like a page awaiting text. Titian's image is one player in a collaged cast, and depicts a scene of violent sexual abduction. In incorporating a scene of transformation and abduction Rauschenberg is illustrating the very thing he is doing with the source. The image has travelled, forcibly taken from one world and entered into another. Rauschenberg's poetics is, like Ovid's, one of mutation and transformation. Here, in the new world, the printed slice of Europa enters into a wider riddle of meaning.

Beneath the red foot there are two intriguing images. To the left, the outline of an empty comic-book speech bubble. To the right, the torso of a diver. Jonathan Katz sees two figures beneath the foot, reading it as two men embracing, identifying them as two divers lifted from a *Sports Illustrated* magazine, one laid over the other, a doubling. He then identifies the traces of an American flag beneath the foot, a direct nod to the most iconic work made by Jasper Johns. As such the two divers become Johns and Rauschenberg. But Ed Krčma doubts the visibility of the flag and argues convincingly that there are not two figures but merely one, cleaved in half. The latter reading feels closer to what is present in the image. The bottom half of the body has been reduced to a blur, but a clear, straight gap can be seen between the two legs. Yet the gap feels less like the space between two bodies and more like a body that has been brutally cut in half and then pulled apart, or as if opened up by a mechanical zip. The arms shimmer, suggesting that the second transfer was shifted just slightly to create a doubling, an echo, the blur of slow-motion photography, but actually recording a different kind of movement, a binary of here, then there, in which the image is laid down, transferred, lifted and then laid down again. The head is more violently shifted, creating the sense of a death mask being lifted off the head of the living. Whether the image is of an embrace or a violent split is hard to be certain, but the motion of the latter seems more likely, the sense of a body being split in two, of this being an act of separation as opposed to connection. The speech bubble, with its emptiness and lack of words, seems pertinent here. A sign which is supposed to house the clarity of language sits empty, as if the body is not granted the function of speech and the clarity of communication that might give, as if in doing so the possibility of direct communication between the body and us has been severed. Or perhaps it is the severance of such a possibility between lovers, a silencing, a body made mute.

In page after page, hovering above the transferred images, are the sounds of the underworld, present everywhere in the silent music of graphic marks. Dashes like slashes, splintered, angular marks eloquently expressing a silent symphony, registering at limits beyond the ear. We are pulled into the echoing swarm of screams and screeches, the marks creating a rhythmical motion, a percussive musical score. It is hard not to see the ghost of Cy Twombly here, Rauschenberg's previous lover. The peculiarities of this graphic language, and their relationship to poetry, music and myth, recall the idiosyncrasies of Twombly's visual language. The hand and its jazz-like motions are an itch, a touch. The hand of the artist on the page mimicking the hand of the lover on skin. Our eye musically traces these marks across the surface in a kind of voyeurism. They portray a new form of desire, the eye becoming a form of touch at distance.

So now we are here, jointly exploring this hellscape, what do we see? What was it you saw? We can view Rauschenberg's works through a political and social lens, particularly in relation to the Cold War. We can view them entirely within the context of formal developments and their context within stylistic and artistic developments in America at the time, particularly in relation to the dominance of Abstract Expressionism at this moment. We can view them through racial and ethical filters, the troubling and problematic ways non-white figures are cast in and into Rauschenberg's underworld. Krčma gives a sophisticated analysis of this problem, concluding that *the fact Rauschenberg selected images of the racial other to correspond with some of the most abject and grotesque characters in Dante's epic arguably signals a degree of unacknowledged ideological complicity.*

There are many paths into these works, but I want to take the path of love, with so much of the groundwork over this already laid by the tender analysis of Ed Krčma. I wonder if we can think of criticism and academia as this, an art history that is not cold, objective analysis, the thinker sat up high offering truth in relation to the work of art. Instead, an art history that is in an intimate exchange with both the artwork and the viewer, where the careful, deep work of critical thinking, of documentary research, often over many years and involving not just critical thinking but intense labour, is an act of faith, love and care. Art criticism might just be a form of love, of opening this up for the benefit of the audience. Love letters to unknown strangers.

In his essay on Rauschenberg, John Cage commented that *beauty is now underfoot wherever we take the trouble to look. (This is an American discovery.)* In context he was referring to the manner in which Rauschenberg appeared to be like a magpie, able to see the beauty and weight of possible meaning in everything, be it Dante or the detritus of everyday life. Yet it fits here, underneath that red-outlined foot, with that split body. Rauschenberg's drawing was made not just in the midst of his relationship with Jasper Johns, but within the context of an America where gay sex was still illegal in every single state. To be gay in America in the late 1950s was to exist in an atmosphere of intense hostility, where the apparatus of the state was used to deny your right to existence. The environment of moral outrage meant it was necessary for Rauschenberg to keep his sexuality private and hidden. The climate of fear in America spiralled into and out of McCarthyism.

As such silence is an essential weapon of defence, the only realistic route to safety. There remains a question, therefore, about whether we should be entering these private spaces at all, whether we should be trying to unpick the relationship of these works to the very private spaces that Rauschenberg seemed to have been protecting. Yet his drawings suggest something more nuanced, a kind of secret safe space which he is inviting us into, with which he seems to be asking us to engage. As if the works had been holding messages and feelings, waiting for viewers to discover them when the world was a safer place. Little love letters from the past, hidden in the depths of the underworld.

In Krčma's analysis of Rauschenberg's earlier work *Should Love Come First?* (*c.*1951) he demonstrates how homosexual desire and love are coded into the piece. He manages to find the source material for a set of footprints in the artwork, lifted from a diagram for a dance routine between partners. This digging out and searching sees many dances take place, between the lovers of the artwork, between the viewer and the artwork and between viewer and artist. The artist, the artwork and the viewer see hands reach out, see us asked to join the other in a dance of love.

Jasper Johns painted *Diver* in 1962–3, as a homage to the poet Hart Crane. In 1932 Crane had jumped, drunk, from the edge of a steamship en route to New York. Reports claim he had been beaten up by a male crew member after making advances towards him. Johns' homage is made up of two identically sized panels, which also mirror each other in marks and composition. The line in the middle of the diptych echoes the split down the centre of the diver in Rauschenberg's drawing. At the bottom centre two hands are pressed into the surface, in motion of a headlong dive down. At the top centre two feet are imprinted, reminiscent of the red outline in terms of their function within the image. Placed at the top of the diptych, facing upwards, they create a sense of a figure stood at the edge of an upturned world, ready to leap upwards, gravity reversed, into the unknown. The work was made only a year or two after Rauschenberg and Johns split, and while it is ostensibly and explicitly a painting about Hart Crane, it seems to reach outwards, to a wider meditation on death and love. Is the diver of this painting the same diver from Rauschenberg's drawing, or is the desire to find clarity of connection an overreach?

I have been trying to find the source for an anecdote I read about Rauschenberg and Cy Twombly, which claimed that when they were together Rauschenberg had taken himself out into the sea to drown, and Twombly had rushed in to save him and dragged him back to shore. I can only find mention of it in a single newspaper article, and wonder if perhaps it is apocryphal. Either way, there is something of water and rescue running through all three artists' work, which seems to speak in various ways of a landscape of love and loss. Yet as soon as you think you can hold it down, can find clarity of what lies beneath the water, it washes away, like a reflection of the surface of a river. Perhaps that is the point.

In one of your Eurydice poems you wrote, *Tonight I dreamt I spilled down into/the webbed chambers of Underworld*. It made me think back to Krčma's description of American life as *the net through which Dante's poetry will fall*. A net, a web: Rauschenberg's transfers are weavings, constructed on a loom filled with the threads of modern life, but used to construct a trap capable of capturing all that and so much more. This was what I wanted my paintings to be, stitched webs, an underworld made not just to replicate something but to capture it. Paintings as webs gathering up everything that might be brought to them. Could paintings be these *webbed chambers*, spaces to house the parts of the self that spilt and scattered out of the world? A chamber implies a private room, and it was the hidden, private parts of connection that I wanted to paint towards.

The paintings were all laid out in the studio, some hanging from the ceiling and the walls and others spread across the floor like huge rugs. It struck me then that they were each a poem. Each of them, in some way was you. Seemingly abstract surfaces, totally free of imagery or figuration, but the picturing of your psychological hinterlands. Each a different space where I might find you, where you might have been, a topography of your internal landscape. Love is the process of trying to get inside the other, while knowing you are viewing the wide expanses of their complexity from a distance. These paintings are pictures of the lover, the loved one and also the gap between.

The medical trial involves fortnightly scans and additional monitoring. The gaps between feel like chasms, both of us waiting for signs of another loss. At six weeks and five days the scans are normal. At eight weeks the sonographer says there is a chance we might be able to hear a heartbeat through the internal ultrasound. At first nothing. Then it comes in with a thump, a racing beat, a visible wave patterning across the screen. The baby's body singing to us from inside the watery walls of your body, a song from the sea.

We hear their heartbeat again at ten weeks, and then at twelve. It becomes a music that steadies our own hearts. At twelve weeks a flurry of tests come back all clear and we find out she is a girl. My first emotion is relief. I had no preference, as far as I was aware, but with this news I think about my experience with my own father, and I recognise a fear of father-son relationships. We are becoming collectors of data, but the only bit that matters is the hearing of her heartbeat, the solid, rhythmic confirmation of her continued existence, of the possibility that she might survive.

Work took me to Australia for nearly a month after the twelve-week scan, and the distance felt impossible. When you went for a scan while I was away I was surprised to notice the pain, longing and jealousy which threatened to turn into a form of anger.

To not hear her heartbeat, to not see her grown, to not hold your hand. My fear of losing her mixed with the terror of missing her solidifying into existence. I was blinded by the longing to see you both, to hear you both, everywhere.

While I'm away NASA scientists release what they describe as the sounds from the darkest corners of the universe. At the centre of the Perseus galaxy, some 250 million light years away, acoustic waves ripple through the gaseous borderspace of a black hole. From the bottomless depths of a devouring plughole come the last gasps and first breaths. The sound waves are so low and stretched out that their frequency is an incomprehensible 10 million years. To make them audible the scientists have had to shift them up fifty-eight octaves to bring them within our range. The sound waves are not just collateral products of the universe's complex machinations but are the thing itself. Vast energy travels through them and enormous passages of heat are regulated by their passage. Whole worlds might be consumed by the black hole, whole clusters of galaxies. This howl is the music of the universe, a great, grand reminder of how infinitesimally small we are.

When I hear it, I'm transported. I see you both there, I hear you both there. The abstract thrum of the black hole emissions takes me back to the rhythmical pulse and oceanic swell of our baby's heartbeat reverberating like a submarine sonar searching for life in the ocean depths. I want to call back, to say I hear you, that I am here.

When you are five months pregnant we move in with your parents while renovations take place at our house. It is one in the morning, a week after my return, jet lag still forming a curtain between me and the world, and you are cramping. You go to the toilet and there is blood. *It's my fault*, you say. *I went swimming for too long, I knew I was too tired.* We call the local hospital, the one where you were born, and they tell us to come in. Bleary-eyed, we drive through the dark.

The hospital seems almost entirely empty, a ghost town. We make our way up to the maternity triage unit, where a single midwife is doing the job of four, a hive of activity. You are asked a series of questions, then led to a bed, and blue curtains are pulled around to enclose us while we wait to be seen. Your ankles and feet stick out of the end of your gown and they seem impossibly beautiful to me, viewing them as my head rests on your chest. The world tilts, and I am reminded of Rauschenberg's red-outlined foot, and his desire to be able to make paintings on fabric so thin that it might not be there, that it might be air. Or what John Cage said about such outlines in Rauschenberg's work, as if they might exist in water or air, as if they had raised his and our feet off the ground. Your horizontality seems not to be a reclining position at all but suspended in air, or water, held at a great height waiting to see if we would fall. Everything is upside down, the air of the room thickening and shifting into a liquid.

Eventually the midwife comes to do further tests. *Let's listen to baby shall we?* This is what we are holding out for, that rhythmical beat that calls from her to us, that says strongly and clearly, *I am here.* The midwife, Holly, says it can sometimes take time to find the heartbeat, but we don't really believe her. It never has before. She runs the doppler across the curve of your belly. Nothing. She shifts position and pressure and keeps moving and searching, but still nothing. The weather of the room shifts. We have seen and felt this shift before, everything getting heavy and thick in the stretched-out silences, in the tiny adjustments of tone and body language.

In this moment I know she has gone, our baby has died, and you know it too. We say nothing. I can see you slipping from me, your eyes glazing, you vanishing inside yourself and your fear and I want to reach in and pull you back but have no idea how. I am slipping too, teetering at some kind of edge, heat rising through my body and my head loosening. We rest our heads against each other, pushing our foreheads together, as if to anchor ourselves and anchor her. *Stay here, come back.* From here I see your feet again, silhouetted now against the blue spread of the curtains. Here it is, the blue of a sky, of a wide ocean, and you are held, waiting to plummet. There are tears streaming down my face and my throat has closed up. My body knows I am drowning, that we are drowning and falling all at once.

There it is. Suddenly, as if from some distant corner, the thumping certainty of her heartbeat. We heard death in that silence, chasing us hard as hunting dogs, but that sound was pure, defiant life. *There. There. Here. Here.*

The midwife has the consultant come and see us to run some more checks before we are discharged. While we wait I lay my head back on your chest, can feel the deep rise and fall of your breath as it settles and the soft thrum of your heart beneath the skin. Adrenaline races through my body, as if I have run a marathon. I am bone-tired from the worry, and collapse asleep on you. I sleep through the rest of the checks. *Like a baby*, you say, smiling, laughing at me, giddy. She is inside you, her heart still beating, and for the moment we have peace.

9

Skin

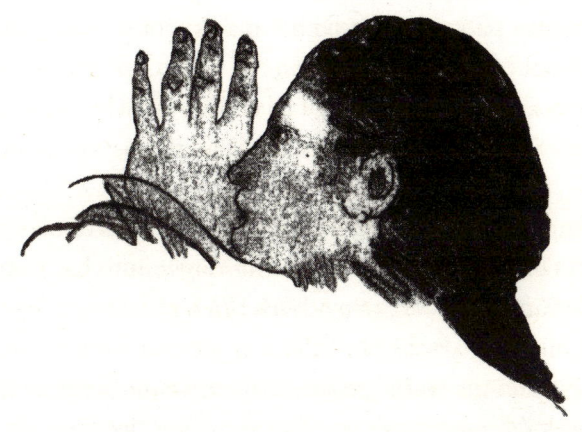

We decide to stop being afraid. Hope takes over, enough to ground ourselves in. I see your body easing, even as your nausea and exhaustion, far from fading, worsen. We hold each moment close, and I begin to feel a small daily grief for how quickly each moment is passing. Suddenly you are showing, with a round firmness beneath the soft smoothness of your belly. I find myself obsessively recording your body, not with any pretence of artistry but with constant candid shots of you, as if I need to somehow make solid each of these moments passing by.

We travel to Venice, in part to see the Biennale and the numerous Titians and Tintorettos. My phone is full of photos of you, standing in front of paintings, against street walls, walking across bridges, lying naked in bed, in the tiny bath in our hotel room. I feel retuned in some way, observant of different details, more alive to the world and to you. I feel a charged desire, and a gravitational pull towards beauty. Everything is heightened.

Most mornings you are bedridden with sickness so I venture off to see a particular painting or exhibition. Even in these short hours I feel a pathetic longing for and severance from you. Two hugely hyped exhibitions among the vast number are by Anish Kapoor and Anselm Kiefer. I visit loaded with expectation, perhaps unfair baggage to carry into an encounter with works of art.

In the accompanying text Anish Kapoor talks of his desire to channel the *dark maternal waters* of Venice into his work. The huge show is displayed across both the Gallerie dell'Accademia and the historic Palazzo Manfrin. The written material about the show says that the works probe at the *limits and materiality of the visible world through works that transcend their objecthood and invite wondrous and sustaining interaction.* Many of them are huge, gooey sculptures and paintings, volcanic eruptions of flesh. Everything is turned up to eleven: the scale, the colour, the visual metaphors. The text talks promisingly about some of the works exploring *the skin of the object as veil between the inner and outer world*. Connections are made of the works' engagement with the folds of Renaissance paintings, of what might happen if edges and contours became diffused spaces of *the possibility to go beyond being*. But it's a Disneyland, the plastic nightmares of a disturbed boy and the promise undelivered.

I have a similar reaction at the Kiefer show, housed in the grand Sala dello Scrutinio, inside the Palazzo Ducale. The vast canvases consume the architecture and decorative scheme of the space. All the traits that I normally gravitate towards in

Kiefer's work are here. Vast landscapes, surfaces covered in thick impasto paint, text inscribed into the surface in great swathes. Huge burnt passages of objects and materials treated with processes which verge on alchemical: a litany of symbols and iconography to decode. Old bikes, shopping trolleys packed with clothes and hay stuck on canvases reaching up to the high ceilings. Views of Venice seeming to glimmer and burn, a nod to the famous fire which tore through this very building. A big metal coffin hovering in the sky of a painting, where trees are made of metallicised branches stuck directly to the fabric. I hate it all. It's nauseating, overloaded in every way and emptied out of meaning. Kiefer's work, which so often taps into the most brutal traumas of twentieth-century Germany, feels suddenly empty here.

The descriptions of both shows talk about light. In the Kapoor, the text says the *subtleties of Venetian light are at play*. The title of Kiefer's exhibition is taken from the writings of the Venetian philosopher Andrea Emo: *Questi scritti, quando verranno bruciati, daranno finalmente un po' di luce* (These writings, when burnt, will finally cast a little light). The vast majority of photographs I take are not of the works of art at all, but of the sheer white curtains hanging over a large window situated between two of Kiefer's huge canvases. Light pours through the fabric, folds breaking the silhouettes of the window panes into a rippled grid across the surface.

In the afternoons, when your nausea has settled, we walk the city, moving from one exhibition to another, slowed by my incessant need to stop and record things, seeing found paintings everywhere, glimpses of visual poetry offered up by the city. It is rarely, if ever, located in Venice's litany of iconic spots, but a beauty that lurks around corners, in alleyways and under lamps. I am not normally a prolific photographer when we travel, and certainly not a good one, but I want to diarise these moments. The underside of a nondescript bridge. Whole buildings melting in the green ripples of the canals. Things appear and things vanish. Even the solidity of the walls is marked by a sense of fluidity and impermanence. Rain stains pouring vertically down, melting the pinks and oranges of brick and marble into darker, seeping reminders of the weather. Edges marked by the rise and fall of water, the green-edged lines drawn on, like abstract landscapes cutting across the often-submerged architectural bases of this floating city. I want to cut out vast swatches of these walls and hang them unchanged on a gallery wall. There are wounds everywhere, cracked surfaces, walls opening up to reveal what lies beneath. A photograph of you in front of some pink plaster, a wide crack revealing layers of worn brick.

The walls of the city are covered in posters for exhibitions mounted during the Biennale. They have become a part of the aesthetic of the place, worn, damaged and ripped, layered to create a collage, a self-perpetuating installation. In one a close-up photograph of a marble statue, abstracted by the waves of the water-wrinkled paper, as if seen through the soft ripples of a river. Even marble melts here. The ecstatic open mouth of the sculpture is a view through the veil of a bedroom. Shadows paint shapes across floors and walls, railings of the bridge patterning themselves like stretched-out wallpaper over the paved floor. Venice, a city built and grown due to its position and role in trade and transit, now literally sinks under the weight of tourism. Yet it offers up other forms of transport between realms. If there was a city for Orpheus to find his way into the underworld, then this would be it.

Venice, famed for its glass mirrors during Titian's lifetime, is a city of myriad reflections. Mirrors appear constantly throughout

Titian's work, and his depiction of *Venus with a Mirror* (1555) in the National Gallery of Art, Washington remained in his studio for over twenty years after his death, the model for multiple versions. The painting is a game of what is seen by whom, what is revealed and what is concealed. Cupid holds a mirror up for Venus, but is she seeing herself or seeing herself seen? Titian's painting partakes in a dialogue perpetuated in the poetry and philosophy of the time that explores the role of the lover and artist's jealousy of the mirror. With Venus as the goddess of beauty and love, the mirror becomes a meta-model of desire. Its magic trick is to never lock down the image, the viewer only ever being able to see that image in that moment.

There are many revelations in X-rays of Titian's paintings, notably how figures are often not fixed from the start and limbs and positions move as the painting finds its final form. What most startles me about the X-ray of Titian's *Venus with a Mirror* – which reveals that a previous composition of a couple standing side by side lies underneath – are the disintegrating forms. The X-ray shows an image scattered in a firework of light effects. Spots of darkness are burnished, breaking down. A shattered mirror has cracks of light everywhere. The looseness of the hand and the brush in the surface creates the effect, when reduced to monochrome, of a body stretched out like light across a pool. An angular burst of iridescent light shows across the face of Venus, her eyes pin-sharp, the act of looking one of the few focused moments retaining clarity. Her hand on her chest barely vanishes into white light. Cupid's legs are in motion across the surface, splashes and streaks of surrounding feet. His body and head explode, rubbed out, erased by great rags of white. Dark curtains and fabrics sit behind, within and over the figures, as if the theatre of the painting is collapsing inwards. I'm not able to read the X-ray technically for information about the painting's history, but see it as a new thing. It presents a possibility of what painting might be, a view into the past and future, a place full of ghosts, an underworld.

Lying flat on our hotel bed, I take a photograph of you standing in front of the mirror positioned between two windows swagged by floor-to-ceiling curtains. The light pushes in at the edges, seems to seep around your body, sculpting it. You are looking in the mirror, hand raised to your hair. A shadow is cast against the wall that you are facing, a shape distinctly you which could vanish into curved abstraction if detached from your image. The curtains frame you, and in the haze of the intense June sun, from the disorientation of my point of view, everything blends together. The photo locks everything into a certainty. In comparison to the flattening one-point perspective of a photograph, looking at you through my own eyes I see an image closer to the X-ray of the Titian painting. The eye travels and collages, more like a painting or a poem. I think of her inside you, her eyes still closed, her world a fluid darkness, her arrival into consciousness formed entirely of touch.

The photographs are mainly of you in motion, walking through alleyways, turning corners, getting in and out of bed. Vanishing around corners, leaving only a fragment of the body in the frame. The following shadow, the curve of your back or wash of your hair. At the Marlene Dumas exhibition at the Palazzo Grassi I take pictures of you walking around the show, standing in front of paintings. In one you are moving from one room to another, the large doorway framed by an ornate marble architrave. Your trailing arm follows the line of the body, the hand turned slightly outwards, the fingers seeming to run across the marble as you pass through. On closer inspection there is a small gap between your hand and the architrave. The hand reminds me of Titian's hands, so often in the process of reaching, but never quite resting on or grasping their target. In the distance is an identical doorway into the next room, a puzzle of entering and exiting, a space that seems to repeat and recall itself.

In photo after photo you move both towards and away from something, in the motion of this transference. Photos of you ascending and descending stairs, a body caught in the in-between place. In most cases your identity is obscured, in part being seen from behind, but also by fragmentation, light and shadows, the movement of your dress. The body becomes a cipher that the viewer of the photograph can imaginatively enter, a site of potential occupation. In some of the photos you have turned back to look at me, to hurry me along. Like Titian's Actaeon, entering from the left, arms, chest and head in the process of halting, wondering, fearing. One part of the body doubting the movement of the other. Your head turned back to return a gaze, to witness a witnessing. The accidental embodying of Orpheus and Eurydice, but flipped. That returned gaze, a threshold between realms reached towards, the site of a doubled death.

At home the photographs continue, in part a diary of your changing body, but also a recording of quiet moments. Photographs of you in the bath, in bed writing, sitting with our cats, getting dressed, getting undressed. Sometimes a suggestion of me, my feet or shadow, is present. The photographs are domestic, intimate and informal, sketches towards sketches, little visual reminders of a moment. Every morning and every night on the way to and from bed we pass what will hopefully be her room. The same room that would have been for the twins, for the others. The light shifts and changes and the window panes are angled rectangles of light across the floor at night. On other days, the red of the cheap curtains, which we have not yet dared to replace in our superstition of readying the room too early, melts into something closer to orange. I capture these plays of transparency, these screens of varying depth and textures. The empty room, waiting to become a nursery, a net capturing these variations, a painting in motion, recording time and sensations. In all these photographs is a mundane monumentality. As source material they are much more open than the knowing theatrics and performative gestures of previous photographic sources I have created. Figures, bodies, moments, spaces and imagery ready to shift realms, building blocks of another world.

I'm in search of an approach to painting that will speak to the everyday miracle of what's happening inside you, and to the quiet moments of beauty that make up love's work. I've spent a career making paintings which are bombastic and where, if there is romance, it's noisy. The losses have reminded me of the grandeur of smaller wonders. I begin drawing you, over and over, constructing an iconography. I was sure that performance would be the generative force, and spent hours in the studio setting up scenes and stage sets but the images feel forced, more like illustrations of destinations. They lack the honesty of the photos and materials I have been collecting.

I print out stacks of the photographs on to thin paper ready to make monoprints. Inking up the glass, I lay down a thin blank sheet of printing paper and place a photograph on top, using the image not as a tight guide but as a source to purposefully disrupt. Sometimes I draw the figure, to remove the context. Other times I select key details to give a suggestion of space or interaction robbed of naturalism. The aim is to untether the figure from the world of the photograph, but sometimes to carry through bits of imagery with it. A doorway drawn in with the minimal number of marks becomes a shape which could slip entirely into abstraction, were it not for its relation to the figure, to that sudden set-up of spatial relationships. I aim for confusions, to surprise myself with these reimaginings of you.

I follow the line of your body in the photo with a pencil, carefully selecting the thickness of the lead, varying the pressure to adjust the amount of ink that might be picked up. Monoprints like this are an exercise in hidden translations, the work of the drawing happening as the ink is pressed into the unseen side of paper. I am as excited by the accidental smudges of ink that get picked up as I am by the intentional lines. The traces of ink across the page create a kind of sheen, a weather in which the drawn images exist. The lines are soft, diffused at their edges. Certain figures and images suggest multiple responses, so I keep riffing on them, working through options. Gradually a cast of characters, symbols and places is building.

Looking for other ways to develop the printed photos, I return to Rauschenberg's method, carefully brushing acetone on to the back of the photo, facing it down on to a fresh piece of paper, then scrawling marks across the back of the paper with no relation to the image beneath. The pressure of the abstract marks pushes the ink from the photographic source on to the paper, creating a net in which an impression of the image is captured. Other photographs I bleach, or rub at with an eraser, trying to push them into obscurity. As with the performance photographs, I am not sure they are images I will use but are suggestions of how I might integrate figures into the network of the painted surface. Printing the photographs on to acetate, I cut them into little rectangles so that they will fit into 25mm plastic frames designed for photographic slides. I layer more than one image, sometimes adding other bits of acetate with drops of ink on. I add acetone to eat at the image, hold some over a candle to melt and meld the layers. Scanning into the computer at a high resolution, I can zoom in so close that even an errant cat hair caught in the slide can suddenly become a thick line drawn across the surface, particles of dust a visible atmosphere. I start purposefully layering in strands of hair, a nail clipping, minuscule discarded bits of the body that might act like forms, silhouettes.

This archive of surfaces becomes the topography of the underworld. Surfaces which indicate mode as much as place, digitised material as feeling. On Photoshop I lay some of the surfaces over the cut-out figures, then vary the opacity so that the figure appears, ghostly within the abstracted world. These were intended as studies, but the digital collages feel like paintings in their own right, pages from a book, story or world that wants to keep generating itself. They feel incomplete without you, as if they need awakening. They need to be the product of collaboration. I need to let them out of my control and into yours. I start printing out your poems, scrawling lines of them on to paper, scanning these in and laying them into the images. Often I will scale the text up so it loses its link to being text, without any direct communication of a letter, let alone a word or a sentence. At other points a line might be visible, suddenly locking words into the image and attaching new readings.

I make physical collages, cutting the figures out of the mono-prints, ripping up paintings on paper, arranging them together on flat surfaces to explore different relationships and combinations. Each iteration suggests another. I am seeking a structural fragility. I want the space of this world to be one of vulnerability. Sometimes a version of you exists within a shape that might have come from you, perhaps the curve of your pregnant belly.

I project the various drawings on to huge rolls of paper. Sometimes a figure, or a fragment of a figure, will become life-size, or even significantly larger. I draw a limb that is eight foot tall, cut it out, sometimes carefully with scissors or a blade, or else ripped to get a rougher edge and to further abstract the form. I create a huge pile of these cut and ripped-out shapes, of bodies, of limbs, of abstract shapes, trying to arm myself with a toolkit made from you which will spiral outside of my control, so that I am merely a medium. I want the paintings to reflect the nature of entering a relationship with you. I feel liberated from the presumptions I would previously bring to the work, free to exist in each moment of evolution, and to let it travel where it travels, in both its lightness and darkness. To paint, and to love, is a journey in companionship, not control.

I can't look towards birth as an inevitability but as a hoped-for outcome of this pregnancy. We are all, you, me and our daughter, in this liminal space of waiting, clinging to the possibility of the light. She is teaching us, in her unknowing state, what it means to occupy the present tense. As the weeks pass you begin a weekly ritual of listing the changes that take place, the staggering developments of your body and of the life inside you as it develops forms of sensation and comprehension. You are outlining the boundaries and limits of the world as she knows it, a world that is all you.

When Titian died in 1576, even he was unsure of his age. Some reports suggest he was over a hundred, and at the very least well into his eighties. He had an astonishingly long life and career, for any period in history. A number of canvases remained in his studio after his death in various stages of completion, with their level of finish a cause of heated debate ever since. In the final decade of Titian's life death was no longer a point on the far horizon but rather one that seemed to stalk him, with reminders of mortality and destruction ever present. Venice was on fire. As Maria Loh identifies, four major infernos wreaked significant destruction and apocalyptic scenes across the city, with major buildings and huge collections of artwork destroyed, starting with the Arsenale fire in 1569 and ending with the vast fire at the Palazzo Ducale in 1574. Earthquakes and floods came to the city, in what must have felt like biblical scenes of destruction. Then in 1575 a great plague ripped through Venice, taking with it nearly one-third of the population. Titian's sight was slowly fading, and touch became an increasingly central part of his painting process. Close friends died, huge wars were fought. He was confronted, within his body and within personal relationships and at a meteorological, political and global level, with reminders of the fragility of life. Commissions due, debts to be chased, taxes to pay, all weighed heavily. The studio as a hermetically sealed space was a myth, with external forces seeping into the conditions in which Titian was working. Death was a presence which crept into his final paintings.

He had been working on *The Flaying of Marsyas* for at least the last six years of his life. The unfinished state of the painting reveals and conceals the uniqueness of Titian's late painting style, the astonishing openness and expressiveness of his brushwork in these final years. Some scholars say that the painting, if completed, would have resulted in a slicker finish, and argue that reading the looseness of his brushwork can be misguided. But even if this were true, the painting is a remarkable insight into the manner in which Titian was developing his canvases at this point. His later paintings demonstrate a career-long fascination with the twists and turns of the hand, where paint is never just a rendering of reality but also a material capable of expressing multitudes, including psychological depth, emotion, light and spirit.

The painting sits in an uncertain place within Titian's oeuvre. Many scholars attribute it, along with *The Death of Acteon*, to the *Poesie* sequence. *The Death of Acteon* seems intended for Philip II and there is a suggestion in letters from Titian to Philip of a second painting, which some speculate was *The Flaying of Marsyas*. Whatever was intended, it continues his preoccupation with Ovid's *Metamorphoses*. Ovid recounts the story of the satyr Marsyas, who challenged the god Apollo to a musical battle on the flute. Marsyas loses and his hubris is met with brutal punishment, his skin entirely flayed from his body.

Titian's painting shows Marsyas hanging upside down from a tree, his body stretching the height of the canvas. To view a figure in a painting larger than life is to shift the function of perspective. A figure which is smaller creates the illusion of depth, with the scale indicating the depth of that distance. A life-size figure means they are pushed right up to the surface to meet us. A larger-than-life figure starts to creep, optically, into the space we inhabit, breaking the presumption of our safe separation. Marsyas hovers and hangs in this space existing in and in between worlds. This is the exact state he finds himself in, being skinned alive, bleeding out, slipping from life to an agonising death.

The painting is claustrophobic, space squeezed out of it. The action is staged shallowly, the dense forest acting as a surround and backdrop, enclosing the drama, pushing everything to the foreground and beyond, to the brink of the surface. It heightens the intensity, creating theatre in which we feel pulled into the spectacle, surrounded by it, not voyeurs of this woodland punishment but somehow active participants. We are made complicit; palpably present. Everything is within touching distance. The forest itself seems alive, not just a decorative backdrop or indicator of place and space but a character in its own right. Such a reading could seem to be Romantic, stretching the limits of possibility; but it does fit with Ovid's text, which suggests Titian is trying to replicate Ovid's imbuing of nature with characterisation. The longest passage of Ovid's retelling is not focused on the musical battle, or the flaying itself. Instead the greatest number of words are given to grief.

The mourners' tears flood into the hungry soil. The earth itself becomes bodily, its subterranean root system described as being made of *deep veins*. The flow of grief is so extreme that a river is formed. A similar anthropomorphising poetics takes place in the painting, where the shimmering passage of leaves seem to come alive, seem to tremble in grief. Paint turned to forest, and forest as participant in the mourning.

Surrounding Marsyas are a succession of figures, some involved in the flaying, some watching. To the left is a violinist, the bow just lifted from the string, the fingers of both hands confirming that this is a sudden and recent arrest of the music. Lips parted, eyes looking upwards, beyond the frame. At the right-hand fringes are three more witnesses. King Midas, in a loose self-portrait of the artist, sitting elbow to knee, hand to mouth, in deep thought as he observes the horror. Below him a dog enters the frame, followed by a toddler that reaches for its soft fur.

John Berger mused on the idea of Titian painting with his right hand while stroking his dogs with his left. Mariah Loh gives the claim solidity and credence, elaborating on Renaissance thinking around the role of pets, where touch is the central mode of communication, where the relationship between a patient and a pet might be one not just of companionship but of connection and deep healing. With the toddler's hand, in stark contrast to the knife which opens up Marsyas, Titian shows the full spectrum of touch's possibilities, able to wound, caress, comfort or heal. Beneath Marsyas is a smaller dog, the type that has appeared in many of Titian's paintings. It hungrily laps up the pool of blood which spills from Marsyas and gathers on the ground. It is a gruesome detail, but exactly what a dog might do. It nods to Titian's earlier Actaeon paintings, in which the hunter became the hunted. But here the body is not pulled apart by the dog; instead Marsyas is forced to contemplate a small animal, inches beneath his inverted, hanging head, taking in what he has spilled out. Stripped of his skin, we are provided with an entrance into Marsyas' open body. In the original text he cries, *Why do you peel me out of myself?* A similar peeling is taking place here, in which we are lifted from our own bodies and placed imaginatively into another. These are the sort of kinaesthetic responses which Titian's late works produce, not just leaps of the imagination and intellect, but felt in the body. Their effect ripples through us physically. Eyes are receptors not just of vision but of touch itself.

The developing role of Titian's hands and fingers in applying paint coincides with the decline in his vision. He uses touch as a crutch to support his sight. For this painter of flesh, there was now no separation between his flesh and the flesh he pictured as he layered on the paint. Our eyes scan across the surface, as if touching it, caressing the subtle shifts and peeling away the buried layers, in an exact reverse. Painting becomes a dialogue around loss, sight, touch and the immediacy of death itself. We are skirting the skin of the other, and ourselves, pressed up against the material limits of our bodies.

How to capture this in my paintings of you? I want to spread everything out across the surface of the painting: the body, the architecture, the landscape, near and far. To bring all depth forwards, opened out, pulled like a skin across the surface. Which of course is what painting does, this twofold paradox of the illusion of depth and the reality of flatness. But I want to push the sense of the distance between these two oppositions closer, or to collapse them together.

The eyes, running across that surface, act as a form of haptic engagement, of touch as being able to move across all these distances at once. For sight to be filled with the distances of desire. Corresponding to the kind of erotic charge between lovers, both bodily in destination and in its ability to run through the body of the viewer. To supercharge the gaps between the spaces of the canvas, both literal space and the space of the content and subject, and that of the viewer. But also, of course, the connecting space of the artist's hand running over the surface and its correspondence, later in time, of the viewer's eyes. Both working in some kind of conversation of distance and proximity. Like lovers.

We first met when I painted you for a play you were performing in. On that day you were all image, and while I had an immediate sense of your beauty there was a kind of emptying of you to an object I had to paint. When we first spoke, at the after-show drinks, there was this immediate charge. You had a magnetism, but also an almost intimidating sense of self-possession. *I like your tattoos*, you said, as without pause or permission you ran your finger across a couple of them on my forearm. *I have a cat paw tattooed on my ankle.* It would be years later that I found out you didn't, that you went the very next day to get it done. One of the tattoos on my forearm was a caricatured doodle I had drawn based on the small dog lapping up blood in Titian's *The Flaying of Marsyas*. The moment your finger touched my skin it felt like an electric charge had been passed through me. For the next few hours, despite the blur of booze, wherever we are in the room there is this intensity and magnetism, every caught glance a confirmation of a shared desire for touch.

I still feel this fourteen years later, and it hits me in surprising moments. At a restaurant in Venice you mop up the last bit of a pasta sauce with a small piece of bread, fold it carefully between thumb and forefinger, place it between your lips with something approaching grace, eyes briefly closing for the final taste. The difference is that now the charge is not just full of the present moment, or the desire for what might follow, but is connected and layered by the entire history of remembered touches between us.

We go to see Mary Weatherford's paintings at the Palazzo Grimani, which are inspired by Titian's *The Flaying of Marsyas*. The building is full of predominantly large canvases, each of a similar scale and proportion to Titian's painting. On first glance they could be described as abstract, tending towards almost muddy swathes of paint dragged across the surface in a mixture of marks, from broad sweeps to splatters and sprays of paint. Attached to each surface are Weatherford's signature neon tubes. They are vertical batons of light, bright-white lines cutting across the surface, casting a stark and distracting glow which bleeds from their edge on to the surface of the paintings. The wires to the tubes are visible, with no attempt to hide the electrical source of their energy and luminosity. As Francine Prose states in her essay on the works, *for Weatherford, the story of neon is the story of modernism in America; it came from Paris, skipped New York, and went straight to California, which happens to be where the artist lives*. It sits in stark contrast to the materiality of the painting. In the openness of its marks and coloration it speaks to the deepest roots of painting, from the undulating walls of cave art to Titian and then onwards to late Rembrandt, Caravaggio, Goya's Black Paintings. Then to the particular expressive potential of mid-twentieth-century American abstraction, in the works of Helen Frankenthaler, Lee Krasner and Willem de Kooning. The presumption of abstraction melts, as the paintings so clearly collect and hold explicit representational ties to a myriad of substances and forms in the real world.

In Titian's painting Marsyas hangs like a vertical wound, upside down, a zip at the centre of the canvas. Weatherford zooms in, unzips the body and spreads it across the entire surface. Ovid's description of the flaying is brutal:

As he screams, the skin is flayed from the surface of his body, no part is untouched. Blood flows everywhere, the exposed sinews are visible, and the trembling veins quiver, without skin to hide them: you can number the internal organs, and the fibres of the lungs, clearly visible in his chest.

No part is untouched. In Weatherford's canvases, touch is given a visual component. The entire skin is spread across the canvas as the eye completes the motions of the knife acting as both tender and violent accomplice. Things that should not be visible are exposed. Weatherford's paintings, alive with movement, tremble with the flow of life forces which, like those veins, we might normally expect to be hidden. They feel incomplete, like Titian's work, but in her case purposefully so. Marks are often alive and rough, as if the painting is still in motion, as if we have been pulled into the drama of the work in flux. Still wet, still being worked. These are opened paintings, pulsing, trembling things.

An astonishing range of colour glows through the brown mass. Splashes of yellow, warm-orange mists soaked into the background. Glittering metallic passages shimmer across the surface, capturing plays of light. Pink and blue stains, dark, shadowy forms and shapes, as if from bodies that might have previously been present. Darkness and light are in constant interplay, bringing the surface to life, creating tonal movement within and across the picture plane. White splatters snow down, red and yellow bursts like the last autumnal leaves holding colour in the mulch. The texture is varied, the fabric of the canvas itself often visible in its weave or the lightness of the fabric shining through, like the last light of day seen through trees in a forest.

These are alchemical surfaces, shifting in front of our eyes, appearing to move between solid, liquid and gas. We are in flux as we watch the site of the painting relocate in front of us. We are floating in the air, we are dragged head-first into the mud, breathless. We are pulled back into flesh, scattered within stardust and then we are debris and silt drifting and pulled along by the flow at the bottom of a river. We are forest, mud, flesh, sky and river. Titian's painting, Weatherford's paintings, take us with them to these primal points between life and death. The dark, watery womb, the growth and expansion, the working towards one such border and an entrance into life, into the world. These are the borders that Orpheus and Eurydice met. To cross the boundaries between life and death, from both sides of the divide. Titian and Weatherford offer up ways in which we might venture towards this in painting.

I stack up a pile of thick paper cut-outs, larger than life-size, in the studio. Each was connected in some way to you and the shape of your body. Some were literal, one lifted from a photograph of you in the bath, which I asked you to take. It shows the curved dome of your belly rising from the water, which cuts a perfect circle around the base. The two even curves of your breasts, shaped into an M, your toes breaking the water. I have also cut out a paper shape based on a photograph taken in the same moment, from where I was sitting in the bath, so the curves are inverted. The shape feels more literal, the body more certain, and the sense of us viewing it from the outside is clear. The photograph you took appeals more, a shape and body the viewer is both outside and inside. The reduction of the body to these few shapes gives it an ambiguity, a disorientation.

I lay a number of the large cut-outs on to the unstretched canvases, which are covered in the marks and surfaces made across the last three years. I rub the back of the paper with linseed oil, to act as a loose adhesive and as a repellent, holding it to the surface of the canvas. I mix up a bucket full of permanent marker, acetone, Payne's grey oil paint, turpentine, cement powder and a syrupy varnish. Pouring it all into an industrial spray gun, I circle the canvas and spray the mixture around the edges of the cut-out, pacing the entirety of the shape, mapping the border of it on to the flattened canvas. I empty out the spray gun, pour in pure acetone and turpentine, spray mists of it at the edge of the thick paint. It eats away at the paint, breaks it down, dissolves it slowly outwards, at first into translucency, and then finally at the outer reaches any trace of the paint vanishes. The paint is not a certain outline, but rather a border sifting from solidity to nothingness. Some of the mixture runs under the cut-out, and despite efforts to keep it weighed down the border is not solid. I lay some weights on top, see some of the mixture of paint and dissolvents pour back out.

Painting is like a dance here, the canvas a stage, and there is no distance between me and the canvas. I can feel it and the paint pushing up against the soles of my feet. I want to record this sense of being present, and to mirror the perspective in the photograph I got you to take of your body in the bath. In this moment I am both painter and subject. I spray around my feet, thinking carefully about their positioning and what this might do to the composition.

After a week the cut-outs are ready to lift. The edges, where the paint is nearly dry, have attached themselves to the canvas. Taking a small, sharp knife, and kneeling down on the canvas, wetting it slightly with oil to help it glide, I slide it under the thick paint-covered paper, the drying paint like a gelatinous skin. Slowly the edges of the paper give way, one skin coming free from another, a slow and precise flaying.

The edges have bled, breaking the contours. Beneath the shape of the body parts abstractions are left, windows on to the layers of the painting largely protected from the thick sprays of paint. The body, or the shape that comes from your body, is now present through its absence, made up of the unrelated array of marks beneath that have been built up over the last few years. Within the curve of what might have been a belly are gridded passages, veins of paint, the silhouettes of materials gathered from the garden and walks. The interior of your body is a wide array of topographies, views onto fractured vistas. There are surprising interrelations everywhere.

I repeat the process, layering up more cut-outs. Sometimes the same cut-out on the same surface, to create repeats and doubles. At other times the images are in exile, finding new homes and relations. It creates more unexpected shifts in scale, where a small hand might sit next to a huge oval lifted from a drawing of your eye. Your body is creating an ever-expanding and self-perpetuating set of estranging formal developments. It is a musical movement between the construction of image and space and simultaneously in the layering and collaging of the deconstruction.

The cut-outs are becoming paintings themselves. Each time they are laid down they pick up more marks on both sides, the surface stiffening. I place some of them on the canvas spread out across our lawn, and connect a power washer, spraying the jet at the canvas. Where the water hits it starts to loosen the paint, and then lifts off layer after layer. I draw with it, leaving impressions and lines across the surface. When the cut-outs are soaked off the canvases they reveal thicker, floating forms on top of the thinned-down, washed-out surface around them. It is another flaying, with water becoming a blade. I want the power jets to create a distance, for the expressive mark to not be linked in these parts by the additions and knowing control and presence of the hand.

Titian worked on *The Flaying of Marsyas* for at least six years, and Mary Weatherford gestated her *Marsyas* paintings for nearly eight. My stack of canvases have now been worked on for over three years, from when we first started trying for a baby. All these surfaces are records: of the physical layers built up, the literal marks laid and the memories of those removed. They record the dialogue between painter and painting, and keep a record of it for the viewer. What lies beneath the skin of the painting is always present in our mind, even when it is beyond us, and we are always in the process of peeling it back, imaginatively reversing the processes. We are archaeologists, with eyes as spades, blades and hands digging through the soil. But paintings made over such long stretches don't exist in a hermetically sealed vacuum. They hold traces of everything happening in the artist's life, in the world that they occupy and engage with. The artist's world haunts the shadows of the work. Paintings become the underworld, the place where the spirts of an age might gather as *thin ghosts*. Even forgetting, like the waters of Lethe, is a form of memory through absence. What might these paintings contain for us? Losses, hope, fears, changes. They are all there. Love, in its constant twists and turns, laid into the canvases at every point. They carry all this and more. Lives which have recorded themselves.

*

At the Mary Weatherford exhibition we take a photograph of ourselves in an old mirror. A black mould-like distortion runs through the glass, not on the surface but in it. It discolours the mirror, but also disrupts the reflection. In the photograph we are obscured. I thought about this kind of moment a lot in the paintings, in regard to Orpheus and Eurydice and in the regular scans of our daughter. We would always speak of the excitement of seeing her, of meeting her at the scans. But of course the scan is never a direct meeting, picturing or seeing of her. Instead it is mediated, the image of her not a reflection but a translation of data through the ultrasound, the technology both a form of connection and separation.

At each scan I have the sense of her getting closer, coupled with an awareness of how far away she is. I cannot comprehend how it must be for you. That sense of proximity and distance amplified in ways which I can only think towards, but not feel into. A form of closeness which will never be replicated when she is born, but that in turn amplifies the strange distance of her not being tangibly present as a touchable, breathing thing outside you. Each time I see her squirming and evolving on the screen, her heart flickering, the sensation hits me strongly. She is growing rapidly, working her way towards existing in the world. We are reading more and more about her development, particularly her arrival at consciousness, and the neurological structures taking shape. Her ability to first become aware of her surroundings and then retain this awareness, to construct and hold on to memory, even if only short-term. It troubles my reading of the pre-birth self as existing in an abyss, as if somehow the mirror image of death. Perhaps it troubles my notion of the state of the self after death.

In *On the Nature of Things* Lucretius writes about the past before our birth:

*The mythical tortures of the lower everlasting time, before we are
born, have been as naught to us. These then nature holds up to us
as a mirror of the time that is to come, when we are dead and gone.
Is there aught that looks terrible in this, aught that seems gloomy?
Is it not a calmer rest than any sleep?*

In the two thousand years since Lucretius wrote this, there
have been huge biomedical advancements in understanding
the pre-birth space, most notably around consciousness and
memory. Yet Lucretius raises still-relevant questions about the
threshold that awaits us before we enter the world and when we
leave it. The image of you and me in the mirror in Venice makes
me think on this, as if it might be closer to the truth. We are
working, in some way, towards this disappearance in death. This
liminal state seems more profoundly present in the late stage of
pregnancy. Our daughter has arrived into her body almost fully
in the third trimester, has worked towards the development of
a self and of a functioning brain, while still reliant on you for
breath and sustenance. A body within a body. Her self-hood as
more than a biological development, is neither fully here and
present in the world, nor is she in a space which is the mirror of
the space after death.

When we look back through the stack of small printouts
of her from the scans she is always blurred. Blurred by the
technology, by the noise of the ultrasound and its ability to
give form to information. Blurred by her motion and by the
limits of the printer. A squirming thing turned into a still
image. The live feed is closer, but still distant, as she comes
in and out of focus. The twists and turns, the blurring of the
image, is something truer to this limbo space of closeness and
distance.

*

Another painting was left unfinished in Titian's studio, likely intended as part of the *Poesie* scheme for Philip II. In *The Death of Actaeon* Diana enters from the left, the foot of her trailing leg cut off by the frame, to amplify the sense of her arrival, in motion, on to the scene. Situated in the foreground, she takes up the majority of the canvas's height, her pink dress bringing her optically further forwards, drawing her starkly out from a painting otherwise made up of reddish-browns and greens. In the mid-distance Actaeon is being chased and devoured by his pack of hungry dogs.

As with many of Titian's other late unfinished canvases, large passages of the canvas are made up of proto-impressionistic loose brush marks. The white dashes of paint tell us that the river is flowing fast. The blurring of paint captures the motion of the dogs as they run. The blur reduces Actaeon from a figure of solid clarity, shows him shifting, loosening, becoming unbodied and working back towards the fabric of the forest and the painted surface. It captures the full drama and metaphysical transformations of a figure violently sent towards his death.

As he worked on them he would have been intimately aware of how near death he was. The unfinished canvases remain locked forever in limbo. The passages of blurred paint are the stages and states of a painting's existence that we do not normally get to see, the curtain pulled back on a process usually preserved for the painter alone. Those blurs remind me of the images of her on the screen, the sense of gathering at the precipice of something leaving one world, something coming into another.

10

Crossings

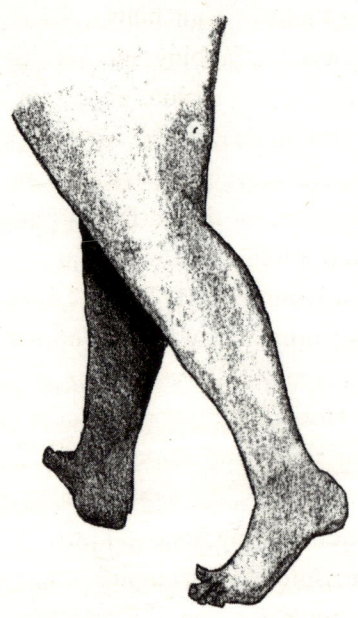

You begin to feel her.

If we reach to the origins of the word *feel* we arrive at the Greek *psallein*, meaning 'to pluck' at a stringed instrument. We find Orpheus, the first musician, his fingers plucking at the strings of his lyre. The instrument could call trees from their roots, could induce forests to wend towards him, could tempt whole herds of animals to his side. During his descent into the underworld, his lyre lulled monsters and beasts to sleep and aroused the deep pity of Hades and Persephone. Here was music that could open the portals of death.

You first felt her at about seventeen weeks. You said it felt *like a snap, crackle and pop*, like little bubbles of air rising. Barely there, only noticeable when you switch your attention to it, in moments of calm and quiet. Then it develops to a flutter, to little butterflies taking flight in your belly. As she grows she starts moving more noticeably, jabbing and kicking at you, stretching you. The force surprises you, and gradually the strength increases and the motions become visible. In these final couple of months you say she feels like a whale, rising from the depths of the ocean, rolling under the surface of the sea, pushing the water into waves, rippling over the curve of its body.

At first I keep missing her. My hand rushing to your stomach just after a kick, waiting and waiting, but nothing. No feeling, no sight of it. But eventually we can feel her push back. We can press in to touch. Her head, her bottom, hand or foot: it becomes clear what is what and what position she is in. She is so close, just the skin of your body, the spread-thinness of your womb, between us and her. Feeling her hand push up, her palm pushing against the pressure of ours, amplifies the proximity and the distance. That boundary is also the membrane of connection. She is so near and so far.

Your skin becomes the site of the connection, of her simultaneous absence and presence. It occupies my every waking thought, and in the studio I think about how to translate this connection into the surface of the paintings, how they might be metaphors of the skin of your belly, with the lives inside the canvas and their relation to the viewer two sides of that divide. Or the artist and the viewer as two sides of this stretched skin. I wonder if in some of the paintings, rather than visualising forms or bodies, absence might be the point. The painting becomes the skin, the conduit through which the figures and lives either side of the divide communicate. It might be the space between two bodies made solid.

We are in the final stages of a slow preparation, readying ourselves for her hopeful arrival. Working through lists of items to order, tasks to do, books to read, birth preferences to decide and write, meetings with our midwife. The closer her arrival, the further it seems between the life we live now and the one we are about to begin. As time shrinks it takes on the shape of another skin. We can imagine a new version of both of us and of her.

I realise how caged I am by my own selfish desires. Even the act of painting will have to alter radically when she is here. I will have to untether myself from the myopia of my inward gaze. I notice it keenly as we begin a series of rituals to prepare for birth, trying to do anything that might keep fear and its attendant chemicals at bay. On the advice of the midwife, we've started perineal massage to reduce the possibility of tears. You are terrified of tearing, but also of the massage, triggering as it does memories of your sexual assault. Initially even the idea of it makes you queasy, yet night by night you find a way to breathe into the physical and psychological discomfort. The midwife suggested it might even be something sexual, yet it could not be further from this for us. But it does feel intimate, deeply so, in a different way, giving over trust to the other, touch as a form of care. You amaze me with your capacity to confront the fears and memories held in your body. It strikes me how your openness to the changes taking part in your body, and the types of bodily experiences you are preparing for, are in stark contrast to my inability to face change.

Immediately after the massage we tend to bathe together, and then I weigh myself. This is nothing unusual, as I tend to weigh myself a few times a day. But it is the absurdity of this act in comparison to what we have just done. A moment of intense intimacy, your body preparing for a transformational experience. This has come after nine months of incredible strain – and more, three years of loss. You have come to terms with the pressures put on your body, embraced this with calmness and grace, even in the moments of distress and discomfort. You felt lost in your body, cheated by it, failed by it. I have witnessed the resilience you showed to trust it, love it, and to empty yourself of the internal and external voices that in darker moments made you doubt it and judge it harshly. You have focused on your body as your home, a place of happiness and hope. I see you do this work, and yet am still locked in the petty narcissism of my habitual struggles with body image. I don't spend time on disgust or disappointment, just feel a profound sense of awe for you. To live in my body is to know nothing of what it means to exist in a body as a site of constant contestation and the requirement to face change.

I compare my desire to keep my body one way to the joy we have both felt in seeing your body change. Squeezing skin between thumb and forefinger, waking every night with anxiety and guilt about what I have eaten or drunk that day. I talk, write and think about empathy, about the desire to try and at least imaginatively step into other experiences and bodies. Yet I am trapped, pathetically and completely, inside my own body.

One day you feel her suddenly tumble inside you. She has dropped, head down, engaged into your pelvis. Overnight your bump noticeably shifts, lowers, the curve at the top flattening out. I think of her inside, feet to the sky, a headstand, her world inverted. Almost daily you get Braxton Hicks contractions, your belly suddenly tightening, becoming solid and taut, the body practising contractions in rehearsal for her arrival.

There is a flood of philosophical writing through history on the existential angst around death, and the ontological unique-ness of the future that awaits us all. Our mortality runs as a spine through our ability to articulate our self-reflections. In comparison there is a relative paucity of equivalent literature on our birth. The philosopher Alison Stone has spent her career researching the links between our anxieties around death and those around birth, specifically our own. In *Being Born: Birth and Philosophy* she muses on the fact that our anxiety about death is its presence as a certain future, the nature of which is unknown. Birth is a past we have all come from, but which is also totally unknown at the level of remembered experience. As she states, *all human beings are mortal and natal.*

If death is a future beyond comprehension, then birth is its mirror. We are unable to recollect this primary experience of coming into the world. The loss of the memory is a primal trauma, the erasure leaving a gap, even a wound. The pro-foundness of this forgetting creates a sense of separation from the self. We know we've had seismic foundational experiences of the prenatal state, of birth and infancy. We were conscious of them, responsive to them, but they are now beyond us. As Stone says, *infantile amnesia means that the rationale for much of our emotional lives lies out of reach.* This distance creates an angst that runs through a life. Stone continues, *when we pay attention to infantile amnesia, we can feel uneasy and uncomfortable realising that we will never be able to make full sense of ourselves ... We are bound in important ways to remain strangers to ourselves.* Self is a stranger.

If death is a final border we arrive at, then birth is quite dif-ferent, and cannot be extricated from what sits either side of it. To know that she is inside you now, that she is conscious and able to hold memories, but just not to store them permanently, is to know that her arrival at this moment of selfhood has come about incrementally. When we began to exist is not a singular moment, a passage we travel through. The arrival into cognition is a slow step-by-step arrival.

She is now full-term, but the profound difference between her experience inside you and when she arrives will be immeasurable. Birth, even if not remembered, is as existentially loaded as death. Arriving must feel like being an alien landing in another galaxy.

I am learning that my interest has been in the space of the divide. The painting as the skin between, the stretched-out threshold that we travel through.

Some of the paintings feel close to completion. I start to arrange them in the studio, think how they might hang together, might be curated within a show and how the conditions of their display alter them. I am still playing with whether to stretch them, locking them into a tight rectangle which will frame them within the perpendicular edges, to be hung flat against the wall. Or whether to hang them loose from the ceiling as double-sided works or stretch them within a frame with both sides visible. I play with stitching multiple canvases together, and in these uneven diptychs and triptychs the focus becomes not the centre of each canvas but the meeting points. The paintings exist along a continuum, operating as a series. Some are seemingly abstract, and some are populated with very distinct bodies. The majority exist somewhere between these extremes. There are contradictions of scale everywhere, the limbs larger than life but buried in the material and optical space of the painting. Yet their scale gives the impression of them floating out of the painting, of operating in the space between the viewer and the canvas, as if they are pressing up against the gaze. The architecture of the painting is full of oppositions and does not hold together. It creates the sense of instability, of the eye lifting the body into multiple positions at once and in many different spatial relations with the view across the screen.

The footprints in one spin me out. The spacing of the steps suggests a tentative move forwards, perhaps even the suggestion of the weight shifting back, a doubt creeping in, a sudden retreat from an edge. The feet remind us of the horizontal pressing on to the canvas, and I see the imagined, invisible occupant of them projecting out from the wall. They are looking down across the void of the gap between the viewer and the canvas, the vertiginous edge of a vast drop into the underworld. It is the space of death and liminality; the horizon line of the painting's imagined space and the horizons of the imaginings of the viewers. A horizon line is shattered and folded to become a net, so that depth and distance are operating in every direction in this unseen, unmaterialised space.

To leap into that figure is to be unbodied, to leave the safety of solid ground and float into the ether, our equilibrium not just eroded but exploded. Gravity is inverted. We exist in front, within, through, down and in the space between us and the canvas. We are simultaneously in imagined, optical, physical and material spaces and situations. It makes me dizzy. It makes me think of loving you, and of our daughter waiting to come into the world. It makes me think of the spaces within you, between us, between you and her, and me and her. The vertiginousness, the dizziness of love.

The majority of our time in Venice was spent at the Biennale, and in particular making multiple trips around the vast exhibition *The Milk of Dreams*. The show is curated by Cecilia Alemani, inspired by artist and writer Leonora Carrington's book of the same name. Carrington is often labelled as a surrealist, but her body of work stretches the limits of such labels. When Carrington's son was small she covered his bedroom in written and pictured stories, often dark, absurd and comic. A boy has ears instead of wings, and sees his head fly off. A box has a box within it and another box inside that, with teeth. A boy eats so much wall that his head turns into an upside-down building. A child befriends a crocodile. Bodies grow other bodies, hybrid animals are not like the ones we recognise but are stacked up like Lego bricks, with the logic of a young child. Some creatures are part machine, part carrot, as if put together like the pipe system of an amateur plumber. It is typical of Carrington's work and career, where everything is subjected to endless transformations. Even in her life there is no splitting of the personal from the creative. As Alemani states, it is a life full of *an endless series of metamorphoses, witch, priestess, visionary goddess, totem animal, a constant transformation that led her to the asylum, to flight, and to exile.* Even the walls of her son's bedroom become the space for wild imaginings, flooding into the domestic space of their home in Mexico City. A bedroom is the place where we travel to dreams and nightmares, where the subconscious is made solid in hallucinogenic projections.

The exhibition is a love note to Carrington, curated using her as a medium through which everything is channelled. In the vast array of her work are a mass of imaginary worlds, a recurring preoccupation with the conditions of the body and its place in an ever-changing planet. The exhibition brings together work from across a huge historical and geographic scope. The text claims: *this means that the exhibition is pervaded by the almost ghostly presence of the past.* More specifically, the ghostly presence is Carrington herself. Instead of presenting a straight chronology, the exhibition offers an ineffable sense of how things rhyme, and how associations are sometimes beyond the conscious reach of the artists involved.

We wander through the vast show taking notes. You are researching a new novel about the life of an imagined surrealist artist, and I can almost see the works physically pouring ideas into you. Something similar is happening to me, this sense where we can't quite trace the lines of influence but can feel the works running through us, shifting thinking and feeling under our feet. It is almost too much to take in.

Moving from artwork to artwork I begin to collect up traces from each, as if echoes of the lives within each are now in exile, populating my memory. From Andra Ursuţa's *Predators 'R Us* (2020) a headless body, arm seemingly cast from a large plastic drinks bottle. Feet sprouting gelatinous-looking tentacle forms, organisms lifted from the bottom of the ocean. Parasitical jellyfish looking to pull the body back to the depths. From Cecilia Vicuna's *Leoparda de Ojitos* (1977), a part costume, part fantastical leopard/human hybrid, one body consuming or colonising the other. A whole host of figures linger from time with Portia Zvavahera's dreamlike canvases. A huddle of part human, mainly owl figures, glowing as if radioactive in shimmering moonlight. Figures within figures, a vibrating orb with a disc-like head has two rough outlines of feet protruding from the bottom. Circumnavigated by a trembling red line, which also traces the contour of the feet. The expanding womb-like torso cocoons an upturned smaller body, both float in mid-air, lifted from the constraints of gravity, feet no longer stuck to solid ground. Everywhere there are bodies joining, emerging from and back into each other, in various states of transformation. Back to where it all began, to Titian's flickering fish, to Ovid's *Forms transformed to bodies new and strange.*

Everywhere the separation of one life from another is

seemingly up for grabs, the borders of self not solid. The same is true of our relationship to Portia Zvavahera's canvases, soft-edged figures, often facing us, with faces either masked or concealed, so we cannot capture their gaze. They see us but we are limited in our ability to see them, in a reversal of the hierarchy that often exists within a painting. They appear to come from elsewhere and there is the sense that they can take us with them, even temporarily. The soft surfaces, the complexity of the figural forms and how they move in space, create the sense that we might be able to just fade into them. That they might be the sites we can travel to, bodies we can enter. We become the figure in the belly, turned upside down, a shadow self, hovering in the ether. But in all these works the opposite is also happening, these figures seeping out of the canvases, lodging themselves into a teeming noise mass of merging bodies which keeps growing as we move around.

Then a moment's rest, and Pinaree Sanpitak's paintings *Offering Vessel* (2021) and *Breast Vessel in the Reds* (2021). In *Offering Vessel* the curved container has a pointed lip for pouring. As such it is an object which can be both filled and emptied. The images retain a sensuality, but in being removed from the limits of the body become functional, mysterious and potentially sacred. They become metaphors for the whole painting, which we can fill with feeling and meaning and which in return can fill us. It is a symbiotic relationship, an intimate form of reciprocal exchange.

This idea of paintings and artworks as containers is opened up in a number of essays in the catalogue, a few of which link back to Ursula K. Le Guin's seminal text from 1986 *The Carrier Bag Theory of Fiction*. Le Guin, riffing on Elizabeth Fisher's anthropological theories, argues that too much focus has been given to stories around weapons as the first human tools. She says:

*We've heard it, we've all heard all about all the sticks and spears
and swords, the things to bash and poke and hit with, the long,
hard things, but we have not heard about the thing to put things
in, the container for the thing contained. That is a new story.
That is news.*

And yet old.

She reminds us that the earliest creations must have been
containers, that even weapons needed to be carried, and that if
we wanted to gather more than we could eat then we needed
something to take things home with us. A found container, a
refashioned shell or leaf or a handmade net or bag. This is how
we create collective sustenance. This is how we stop things –
seeds, ideas, words – escaping and hold on to them into the
future. She reminds us of the ways in which this gathering, containing and carrying then unfolds. How the home, the museum,
the sacred shrine become large models of the container.

This expands fluidly into the nature of storytelling itself. The
work of art, the novel, can be seen in this context as containers
that carry. Devices in which information, story and feeling are
carried collectively forwards in the cultural memory. She suggests a reconfiguring of both the history and narratives, around
containers as opposed to heroes and weapons. While conflict
might drive aspects of a novel, it is limited compared to the
vessel. The vessel can carry conflict and harmony, *since its purpose is neither resolution nor stasis but continuing process.* She cites
Virginia Woolf's glossary, where heroism gets defined as *botu-
lism*, as Le Guin puts it, *And hero, in Woolf's dictionary, is 'bottle'.*
She proposes the bottle as the hero, the vessel which contains,
holds and carries something else forwards. She situates this as
the primary driver of the novel as a form. A book is a natural
container, as she says, *A book holds words. Words hold things.*

She sees this act of carrying as spanning across time and space, the means by which humanity is collectively threaded together. This is *how people relate to everything else in this vast sack, this belly of the universe, this womb of things to be and tomb of things that were, this unending story.* The universe becomes embodied, a great wide belly. The womb and the tomb are the ultimate symbolic carriers of future possibility and past states. But there are *arguments of some feminist critics against symbolising the female body as a container – specifically, one for carrying children.*

The problem, it seems, comes if we think of the female body as passive, as if there is not agency. This does not sit with my impression of the relation between you and our daughter. You are carrying her, but the boundaries between the body as container and the being growing inside aren't solid and the relationship works in both directions. You are both contingent, both in the entire process. This dissolving of the boundaries seems to be a model for ideas about the self. Only the pregnant body has occupied both sides of this experience. I have seen how she has grown and changed inside you, but also how she has already changed you, me and us. Carrying is a form of love as collective exchange and growth.

Donna J. Haraway's catalogue text expands upon all of this, arguing that models which claim that organisms, be they cellular, bodily or societal, can be *self-forming and self-sustaining* are *fantasies.* The same being true of claims applied to the work of art as an autonomous object, able to exist without interaction in its production or consumption with the outside world. She argues instead for what she calls *a carrier bag for ongoingness.* That is, models of living and artmaking which come about through *making-with*, through complex webs of interactions. As she says, *nothing makes itself*, embracing the interconnectedness of all things and the idea of mutual collective growth. This is exactly what it seems is happening to you during pregnancy, at a biological, psychological and philosophical level. A joint journeying.

I carry all this back to the studio. We are edging ever closer to your due date, so I am wary that I will be covered in toxic paints just at the instant your waters break. The stolen moments in the studio see me become a viewer rather than a maker, and this brings a surprising clarity.

The studio is overflowing with material. The large canvases hang on the walls, each a portal into a view of the underworld, into a landscape of you. The still-unstretched canvases, some stacked, some laid out on the floor, some hanging from burnt bars from the ceiling. They are curtains, stages and divides. Stacks of paintings on paper, thousands of them, like unbound pages from an illuminated manuscript. Printouts from the filmed and photographed performances, drawings, the cut-out paintings, the books. The little cardboard box paintings, like stage sets for plays neither written nor performed. The shift in scale creating all kinds of different entrances, or thresholds to be imaginatively crossed.

They are various forms of containers, many of them seemingly emptied out. The books have their middle removed, the stage-like sets are empty of action, the paintings appear less to be populated by living bodies and more by the echoes and traces of past lives. They are containers awaiting your arrival, invitations for participation. Portals to chambers of the underworld. I am brought back to Ovid, back to Orpheus and Eurydice, back to you and your poems. The entire mass of works together forms a poem, each object in this disordered space a stanza. The word 'stanza' literally translates to mean room, and all of these are rooms to enter, or to stand at the precipice of entry. I suddenly realise that the artworks are not destinations in themselves, but closer to works of architecture, waiting for the viewer to explore, to become the central protagonist of a shifting drama.

They are, then, not so much of you but for you. Ready for you to open them up further, through looking, through language. For this engagement to be a form of poetry, of writing from and into the surfaces, populating them. It is a reciprocal relationship, one close to the movements of love, existing not in one or the other but in the space between. Perhaps I always got it wrong, thinking I could depict an underworld. Perhaps the underworld is this space between, be that between lovers, artist and artwork or viewer and painting. A great wide chasm, infinitely wide and ever expanding and utterly ethereal. These relationships are of exchange, deep empathy.

On a visit to the studio, you ask me which are the final art-works and which are studies, and I cannot answer you. Later I realise that there is not a hierarchy between studies and final works, or even between the objects in the studio and everything else. All these containers are porous, both gathering and spilling meaning into and out of each other. The artwork is an under-world capable of holding everything, even if some of those things remain hidden and secret to many, or part of a private engagement.

Le Guin's essay finishes, *still there are seeds to be gathered, and room in the bag of stars.* This is the work of art: a carrier of seeds, seeds which are then sown and grown and populate imagina-tions. We then carry these with us, these seeds, beyond our encounters. The possibilities become dizzying because they are as infinite as a sky full of stars.

It is 1575 and Titian is deep into old age. Outside, Venice con-tinues its ceaseless flux of trade, the churn of people, goods and ideas flow into, from and through this city, this economic and cultural hub of Renaissance Europe. Yet the lifeblood of its success was also the reason it was so susceptible to the influx and spread of disease. Among the many arrivals that summer was the plague. Despite the lessons learnt and the systems developed from previous instances the authorities are slow to act, the stagnation the result of the noise of conflicting expertise and concerns over economic impacts. The wealthy flee, the poor are left, trapped and waiting, the city is cut off. Over the next two years nearly a third die of the disease.

Titian is still working in his studio, stacking up the paintings, deciding which to declare finished. He has begun work on a large canvas, a painting of the Pietà. Early biographers seem certain the painting was intended for the altar of the Capella del Cristo, where Titian wished to be buried. It is confirmation that Titian was not just, of course, aware of his mortality but that he was thinking deeply about it. In the bottom right-hand corner of the painting is an ex-voto, a painting within a painting. The small canvas depicts Titian and his son, Orazio, praying to Mary, and is widely read as signifying a plea for her to protect them from the plague. The painting itself becomes both a prayer and a protector. Titian turning to paint in the hope that he can pull off one last magic trick, that this might be his shield, that it might hold disease and death at bay. After a year the plague finds its way into Titian's life. First his son succumbs, and in August 1576 he himself dies, officially from a fever. Due to the plague his body cannot be transported to his hometown of Cadore in the mountains, so he is lifted through the disease-ridden streets to the Frari. The painting, the protector turned memorial, remained unfinished in his studio.

The painting now hangs in the Gallerie dell'Accademia in Venice. The action is staged at a shrine, centred on a domed niche, a split pediment flanked by stone columns and two stone statues, one of Moses and one of Sibyl, atop plinths with a lion's head carved into the front of each. All the figurative action takes place in front and within this setting, the architecture acting as both a surround and a backdrop, the figures arranged in the bottom half of the picture. In the centre is Mary, with the dead Christ lying across her lap. To their left the grieving Mary Magdalene, with a putto angel in the bottom left-hand corner. To the right, kneeling in front of Christ, St Jerome. In the top-right corner is a glimpse of a dark night's sky, the scene cloaked in darkness, only illuminated by the flickering light of flames.

St Jerome wears a face clearly identifiable as a self-portrait. His hand reaches out to Christ's, into the shadows. His face is upturned, looking into the dead Christ's face. Here, Titian is present in disguise, both there and not. The hand and the eyes in a haptic engagement with the corpse of Christ, the artist and St Jerome, in the same body, in grief, their touch and sight reaching into the both infinitesimally small and infinitely deep gap between life and death. It mirrors our witnessing, but even more so mirrors Titian's mode of painting. Fingers loaded with paint pushed the substance directly into the fabric, removing the distancing effect of a brush. To paint flesh, to paint the body, to work paint into both the representation of the living and the dead, to operate in the space between.

The figure of Mary Magdalene arrives from the dark. Her right hand is raised in halting despair. She looks out of the picture frame to the left, her mouth open, her eyes dark sockets, a mask of grief. She is in motion, her left foot crossing the front edge and step of the shrine, taking her to the very edge of the painting, to the step from the illusionary space and towards our space. She is in the process of passing from one world, one state of living, to another.

The paint holds light, literally, through a manipulation of

the physics of the materials. The skin of the body is glazed and varnished, meaning that light pierces these tinted transparent layers, is devoured by the darker passages, then reflected and refracted by the array of marks. The marks act like a net, catching some of the light within the material, leaving the rest to pour out of the surface, from within. It means the surface of the body, of the painting, of flesh itself, is suffused with light, which is both captured and released, which both enters, exists and leaves its traces within the surface. The body of Christ becomes a wound, open to and pouring forth the light of God. Above the body of Christ, in the dark shadows of the domed niche, is a vibrant dappling of light, which seems to be more extreme than we might expect was the seen one of naturalism. It draws the eye, creating a balance and rhyme with the light coming from the body. One below, one above, as if the light has escaped the body and risen up, is sat here, unbodied, floating in the air.

It is alchemy in action. It is the sort of handling of paint that Titian had spent a long life evolving and perfecting, reaching its apotheosis here. It is paint as a sign capable of having a multiplicity of reverences. It is paint as the metaphorical carrier bag that Le Guin mentioned. Paint here as itself, paint as becoming flesh, as containing spirit.

I find myself so close to the painting that I can almost see my breath fog over the varnish, can feel a desire to reach out, to push my finger at the surface. Scattered across the whole painting is a spider's web pattern of cracks, where the varnish has given way to expansions and contractions, splitting like the bed of a dried-out river. The varnish sits as the final layer on the painting, a layer that brings everything together, that acts like an almost invisible sheen of liquid glass, a hidden, vanished unifier, finisher. It places the entire thing behind this only-just-there curtain or window. But a varnish doesn't sit separate to the paint, it gathers in the undulations, skimming over the risen patches. Here those cracks bring it back to visibility, back to the attention of the eye. It reminds us of the lie of art as permanent, of the fact that this thing is material, will degrade and rot like the rest of us, that it is slowly being pulled apart, still holding on.

We are in the strange final days of the pregnancy; you are waiting for signs from your body. We have been working on breathing exercises for the labour and you have this vision of each breath taking you closer to meeting her, like curls of light entering and then leaving the body, rising up and clustering together in the sky, like a vast and growing, swirling equivalent of the Northern Lights. In bed at night, we practise breathing deeply and I try to paint the picture with words, to help set the rhythm of your breath. While I can't see her yet, I can see a vision of your breath made solid, and I feel in that moment a lightness and excitement, that it is all going to be all right.

When we first started trying, we wondered about what it meant to bring a child into this world and its escalated spiral of doom. How to bring something into the world in its end days? I wonder if art can help, if painting might offer a route into touch and connection and might be a reminder of beauty. Might paintings be part of that effort to reach out into a shared collective? Beauty, so often seen as soft and decorative, is a route to wonder, and the hope of healing. Perhaps my desire to depict the underworld is not about painting a view into death and loss at all, but rather the other way: a view back out to the light, towards the future. Not empty stages, but full of the unbodied voices of the collective. Not a view into suffering, but into the great expanse of a shared sky. When she is here, I want to show her that, if nothing else.

We read about oxytocin, a chemical produced by love, safety, sex. This chemical triggers labour and helps it progress. If you shift into a state of fear or panic your body will produce adrenalin, and the science seems to suggest that this either flushes out the oxytocin or even inhabits and blocks the continued production of it. We think about the ways in which we can create an environment in which you are able to stay present, calm and feel safe.

You are not worried about the contractions, or surges as the books tell us to call them. You are worried about the *fear* of the pain flooding in, and about losing control. That the birth might become a trigger of previous traumas. We focus on things to keep you in the moment, to hold fear at the door: music, touch, breath. One night it arrives unexpectedly, as fear often does.

The first I know of it is as an incursion into a dream. Your voice, a cry in the distance, seeping into my sleep. Slowly your voice comes closer, pulls me back into the bedroom, into wakefulness. You aren't next to me, and it takes a moment to realise your cries are coming from the bathroom. Your voice is weak, but desperate. I stumble through and find you collapsed on the floor, circled around the toilet. I can hardly make out what you are saying, you are limp, barely there at all. I try to lift you into my lap. You can't keep your head up, can barely open your eyes. You are trying to tell me something but your speech is slurred, I can just about make out you saying, *I'm losing her, I'm losing her*. There's no blood but I call 999 and, tears streaming, desperately try to keep you conscious, worried that I'm losing you. *Stay here, stay with me, stay here, stay with me*. The wait for an ambulance is going to be too long, so they tell me to get you to the hospital.

I half lift, half drag you from the bathroom, across the landing, down the stairs. It takes more than fifteen minutes to travel this short distance. You are violently sick several times. I manage to get you to the car, your legs jelly. As we drive to the hospital my vision is smeared by tears, I look across to see you unconscious, head lolling to the side, eyes rolled back. I fear pre-eclampsia, a stroke or a brain haemorrhage, like your grandmother died from young. I park at the entrance to the women's centre, grab a wheelchair, drag you into it. An ambulance comes blazing up behind us, a sudden rush of lights and bodies as they pull a patient out of the back. I press the button for them to open the doors, signal for the paramedics to go ahead, but after one look at you they insist we must go first. I can barely steer the wheelchair. We are rushed into a room in the EPAU unit and a couple of nurses help me lift you on to a bed, and suddenly there is a flurry of people in the room, gathering information from me, taking your temperature, your blood, checking your pupils. In minutes you are on a drip for fluids, a monitor around your belly to check the baby, medication being run into your body through a canula. You are awake again, continuously sick, listing to the side, slurring.

The initial activity seems to stabilise you. Then there is a rhythm that settles, a movement from passages of waiting to bursts of arrivals, activity and tests. Notes are taken, conversations had in corners and a drip feed of information delivered. They seem happy that you and the baby are stabilised, and have now started the diagnostic process. In the spaces of waiting, we struggle to hoist you on to a bed pan, your head still lolling. You are now more conscious, just about able to talk, but as if very drunk, half asleep. One of the doctors comes in to let us know you are being taken for an MRI on your brain. In the wait for the hospital porter I watch the little printout from the machine you are plugged into, graphs of data tracking our baby.

We lift you on to the wheelchair and I follow as the porter wheels you for your scan. It is a twenty-minute walk, through many doors, corridors, a freezing-cold bridge which joins two parts of the hospital and up and down several elevators. The sudden scale of the hospital reveals itself, all these lives. On the way I notice several people looking at you, and the look in their faces, somewhere between pity and concern, terrifies me. *What if this is where you die? Where you both die.* I picture our house, wandering around alone.

In the depths of the hospital you are wheeled up to the double doors of the scanning room. We wait. Your speech has improved a bit. *She'll be okay? I'll be okay?* I hold you tight, breathe in the smell of your hair and we cry into each other. The lights above the door go from red to green, a signal for me to wheel you in, and we lift you on to the conveyor bed, ready to be funnelled into the scanning tube. I kiss you on the forehead, blindly promise it will be fine and head outside. The doors shut; the lights go from green to red. A couple of doctors go into the adjoining room, where I can see a huddle of them around screens, presumably waiting and then looking at the images of your brain. The doors close and I resort to pacing, counting, closing my eyes and attempting to imagine myself elsewhere.

Red to green. Doors open. Everything in reverse. Lifting you back on to the wheelchair, waiting for a different porter. It is his first day so on the return journey we get lost several times. Back in the hospital room we wait, you are given more anti-nausea meds, there are checks on your drips and canula, the dance we have started to perfect with the bedpan.

Towards the end of the day a new doctor comes to see you. They have been able to rule out a vast number of things, including most of the particularly worrying possibilities. I feel the fog lift. They are still unsure what it is, and want to keep you in overnight to run some more checks. We are moved to another room on the sixth floor, with a little pull-down bed in a cupboard where I can sleep.

You are wiped out. I have been taking lots of photos, in part to pass the time and to avoid my brain overthinking. Photographs of the room, of the blue curtain across the window, of the way the light breaks through the material, shadows casting shapes on to it, as if figures or objects just the other side of a divide. Then the view outside, to the great spread of illuminated windows, each a little cell, an opening on to another life, the sweeping feeling of sonder multiplied. The view of a long corridor, the angle from up high cutting the figures who pass through into just sets of legs in motion. Everything in transition, the hospital as a living, pulsing organism.

Most of the photos are of you, of your feet popping out of the bedcovers, or your hand resting on top. Or the machines and tubes you are linked up to. The body, when reduced to fragments, shifts. The legs in the photos look as if they could be from a body floating, drowning, rising or falling from a great height. The blue light which floods the room through the curtains suggests something of the light beneath the surface of an ocean swell.

Your condition has steadily improved overnight, to the point where you seem close to your normal self. Slowly the doctors have been able to rule out many things. They are still not sure what the cause was, but they suggest it might be viral labyrinthitis, a condition that can cause the type of dizziness, vomiting and other symptoms you had. They suggest that this, combined with late-stage pregnancy, could have resulted in a particularly severe episode. One of the main symptoms is vertigo, which the doctor said might explain why you had been unable to stand or hold your head up. The entire equilibrium in your body disrupted, as if the virus had taken you to the brink of an invisible and vast drop. The labyrinth describes two parts inside the ear, one of which is a complex network of channels filled with fluid. The loss of balance comes from the interruption of these channels.

Things settle by evening and soon we are home. The very next day you agree to a big family meal at our house, despite my resistance. It is as if no one realises quite how serious things were, or how precious and precarious these final days are. No one else saw you, head lolling, heard you begging me not to let our baby die, not to let you die. That night I sit in the corner of our shower, weeping and terrified.

The morning after we get home, you begin to experience false labour for a few hours each day between 3 and 8 a.m. You are so close. We are so close to meeting her. You move between the bed and the bath, finding comfort as always in water. Then, five days after our return from hospital, your waters break. You stand by the bath, the cats at your ankles, all of you looking at me confusedly. Another bath, and the contractions increase in intensity and regularity. *It's started*. We call the hospital and they say to come in. We go through our tick list of things to gather and drive there. We are in the midwife-led unit and after an inspection and assessment we are told you are not yet in established labour. They offer a room on the sixth floor, where we'd stayed during our last visit. You are afraid, anxious – *I want to go home*. They agree that's fine, and tell us to wait until the pain is severe.

You get straight back into the bath, and our cat Luna all but climbs in with you, perched on the thin lip by your head. Your parents arrive, and your dad makes you a vast bowl of pasta which your mum and I feed you between contractions. From the bath you text my mum, a few close friends, my sisters. I see the comfort you get in surrounding yourself by this chorus of female voices, all united in telling you: you have this, that it will all be all right.

Over the next few hours the contractions increase until you are at the point where you cannot speak. Your breaths become harder but you hold on to them, gripping my hand tightly, your mum stroking your hair. We hold off a bit further, wary of being sent home again, and then eventually it is too much for you to bear and we head back to the hospital. They confirm it: not long now. She is on her way.

Later you'll ask me what I remember, and what I say is not accurate at all. I recount the moments as if the memory of them followed the linear flow and rhythm of time, merely a succession of events. The truth is, from the moment we enter the hospital time scrambles.

In the main what I remember is you. Everything else falls away: the walls of the birthing suite dissolve, the midwives and your mum behind a fog, my own body absented. Things shift in and out of focus, made real only by the parts you touch. I'd like to say I was thinking of her, thinking of the magnitude of the journey she was undertaking, that primal shift, but for me everything is you.

You're on the floor, breathing, gas and air pressed to your mouth. We are counting, your mum's and my voices shaky and out of time, holding you, trying desperately to keep you in the moment, in your body, in the room, when every part of you wants to escape it. Blood on your thighs. The strain in your neck. Your hair tied back, strands escaping across your collarbone.

You are in the pool, limbs white underwater, my arms under yours holding you up, our faces inches from each other. The space between us is what I remember, that is what I feel and see. The gap has almost vanished, not just physical proximity but the kind of melting effect of love. On the other hand it is a great wide chasm, and I see you at the far corners of it, undergoing the kind of transformational experience that I can't comprehend. You are lifted by it, above me, and in your eyes I see this look that says *you have no idea.* I don't. I am there but absolutely not there. I cannot picture the vast and endless bodily and embodied landscape of birth. Everything else is outside it, it is all you, and all her, and everything else is the other side of a great divide, merely calling across the border.

Then suddenly, from the hellish panic of transition onwards you are elsewhere, you are transformed, more powerful than I have ever seen you, reaching somewhere deep and beyond. I remember talking into your ear, and for the last time through you to her, saying I love you, you're nearly there, you're nearly here. Then in one push, you are, she is. Crying: all of us, your body shaking with laughter, your eyes wild and present as the midwife lifts our daughter on to your chest.

Everything up to this point seemed to happen at once. The entire birth, from the perspective of witnessing it, was a kind of rupture in time and space. The experience a painting is able to hold, many moments in one frame. Now time regains itself and crystallises into distinct, singular moments. Her turning from grey to pink, eyes black and wide open. Her curled body against my chest as you deliver the placenta. Her dark hair drying into curls as she drinks from your breast. But most of all, there is the first night and morning together. The blue room.

It's captured in my favourite photograph. The early-morning light is pouring in through the semi-transparent blue curtains, the entire room drenched in this blue glow. Our daughter is on your chest. The mundane miracle of her having been inside you a few hours ago is beyond me. Here you are both bathed, submerged in this blue. Your tired, elated eyes look straight at me, past the camera, into mine. Your hand is cupped around her tiny head, her profile half vanished into the shadow of her face across your chest. Even the white hospital sheets are blue, everything existing in this magical underwater world. It is as if the instance of her birth has chucked us into this altered version of the world. For all this time I had been thinking about underworlds, about different worlds to enter, explore and find you in, to find her in. Yet in her arrival the world itself unlatches and reforms, drowned in beauty.

It is nearly two years to the day from when the twins would have been born. On their could-have-been second birthday you sit beneath the painting I made for them, our daughter suckling, and I think of the other possible paths. The losses, the waiting, the pain, the love. The version of them and us existing in parallel universes. I swear that if I shut my eyes I can feel them, can see them, can feel it all. As if all those scattered selves of us and you and them are somehow floating like charged atoms in the room, like a painting's palimpsest, every mark existing even if it is unseen. It is something close to a secular sacred moment, something spiritual in the ether.

She is here, you are here, we are here together. If I close my eyes I see you, arriving from deep water, from a place no light can reach. You are swimming upwards, seven flickering fish alongside you. Light starts to work its fingers towards you, scattering, stroking your shoulders and hair. Higher, and the fish fall away until there is just one that rises with you, silver and perfect, certain in the gathered light.

Notes

Chapter 1: Splitfish

p. 2   The quotes *'Forms transformed ...'* and *'for ye have changed ...'* come from Ovid's *Metamorphoses*, in the English translation by Arthur Golding (Macmillan, 1965). Both are taken from the opening four lines of Book 1.

p. 5   *'lifeless to the ground'* is from Book 10 of Ovid's *Metamorphoses*, in the English translation by Mary M. Innes (Penguin, 1955), p. 225.

p. 5   *'rouse the sympathy of the shades'*: ibid.

p. 5   *'thin ghosts'*: ibid.

p. 5   *'love was too much for me'*: ibid., p. 226.

p. 5   *'weave again Eurydice's destiny'*: ibid.

p. 6   *'straining to clasp ...'*: ibid.

p. 6   Ann Wroe's suggestion, that Orpheus' first note might contain all of music, comes from her extraordinary and inventive biography *Orpheus: The Song of Life* (Jonathan Cape, 2011). It has been key to shaping my thinking around Orpheus.

p. 7   For more information on the National Gallery's exhibition *Titian: Love, Desire, Death* go to the exhibition catalogue of the same name (National Gallery, 2020). During the opening I was also indebted to the observations of three leading Titian academics: Professor

217

Martin Kemp, Professor Paul Joannides and the curator of the exhibition, Dr Matthias Wivel.

p. 9   The context around the commissioning of the *Poesie* paintings is amalgamated and cross-referenced from various texts, including *Titian: Love, Desire, Death*, *Titian* by Filippo Pedrocco (Rizzoli, 2000) and *Titian* by Charles Hope (Chaucer Press, 1980).

p. 9   Thomas Puttfarken's *Titian and Tragic Painting* (Yale University Press, 2005) has the most convincing and comprehensive account of the eroticism in Titian's *Poesie* paintings, and more pertinently Philip II's intense erotic engagements and intentions.

p. 11   I first encountered Florike Egmond's research on the sixteenth-century natural history drawings and watercolours of fish in her *Guardian* article, '16th century "zoological goldmine" discovered – in pictures' (9 March 2017). Further context and information were given in an email exchange, and then in her book *Eye for Detail: Images of Plants and Animals in Art and Science, 1500–1630* (Chicago University Press, 2016). It was my exchanges with Florike, and her patience with my flights of fancy, that made me realise that Titian's fish is clearly not a chromis fish at all.

p. 13   '... *and lest some part might be bereft* ...' comes from Book 1 of Ovid's *Metamorphoses*, in the English translation by Arthur Golding.

p. 13   '*My soul is wrought to* ...': ibid., opening lines.

p. 14   '*Art cannot be fixed* ...' is a quote from Siri Hustvedt's collection of essays *Mothers, Fathers and Others* (Sceptre, 2021). The quote is found on p. 190; it is the final paragraph of her essay 'Living Thing' (2019), which explores the ways in which a work of art inhabits the viewer, both during and after the encounter.

Notes

Chapter 2: Step

p. 21   '*There are more secrets ...*' is a quote from *Julia and the Shark* by Kiran Millwood Hargrave, with Tom de Freston (Orion Children's Books, 2021), p. 1.

p. 23   '*strays with aimless steps ...*' comes from Ovid's *Metamorphoses*, Book 3, in the online English translation by A. S. Kline. Here and elsewhere, the rest of the recounting of the story is a paraphrasing of Ovid's account.

p. 24   '*tell, if you can ...*': ibid.

p. 24   '*His dogs catch sight of him*': ibid.

p. 24   '*Greedy*', '*Savage*' and '*trusty*': ibid.

p. 24   '*The whole pack gathers ...*': ibid.

p. 24   '*a wordless head*': ibid.

p. 24   '*He might wish to see and not feel*': ibid.

p. 24   Various books on Titian have been key to shaping my engagement with the works, the ways in which I think about them and look at them. Some have been particularly pivotal. Thomas Puttfarken's *Titian and Tragic Painting*, with its interrogation of the translation of tragedy from literary and poetic conventions to painterly ones, Maria H. Loh's *Titian's Touch* (Reaktion Books, 2019) for its exploration of touch in Titian's painting and the haptic experience for the viewer, and Rona Goffen's *Titian's Women* (Yale University Press, 1997) for its exploration of the male gaze in Titian's painting of the female nude.

p. 25   Accounts of Philip II's knowledge of Ovid are written about in most books on Titian. Charles Hope's *Titian* and Thomas Puttfarken's *Titian and Tragic Painting* were my primary sources. Puttfarken's book deals particularly well with the intimate nature of the encounter between Philip II and the *Poesie* paintings.

p. 25   '*aimless steps*' and '*strange wood*' come from Ovid's
         Metamorphoses, Book 3, in the online English translation
         by A. S. Kline.

p. 25   '*sacred grove, a cave mouth dampened*': ibid.

p. 26   David Rosand's ideas around *colorito* as a verb are
         explored in depth in his essay 'Titian and the eloquence
         of the brush', in *Artibus et Historiae*, Vol. 2, No. 3 (1981),
         pp. 85–96.

p. 29   '*you should have looked at me*' is a quote from Patience
         Agbabi's poem 'About Face' (2012), which was published
         in *Metamorphosis: Poems Inspired by Titian* (National
         Gallery, 2012).

p. 33   '*My soul is wrought to*' comes from Ovid's *Metamorphoses*,
         in the English translation by Arthur Golding. It is taken
         from the opening four lines of Book 1.

Chapter 3: Breath

p. 35   The *Collins Online Dictionary* was the main source for the
         research around the etymology of the word 'fold'. This
         is where the quotes '*become doubled upon itself*' and '*give
         way . . . fail*' are taken from.

p. 35   The ideas around embryological development
         were collated and cross-referenced from various
         sources, including the Wikipedia article on 'Human
         embryonic development', Tom van Gelder's website
         Phenomenology and the journal article 'Human origami:
         The embryo as a folding life continuum' by Glenna
         Batson, in *The International Journal of Prenatal and Life
         Sciences*, Vol. 01, Issue 01 (July 2017).

p. 38   The photographs from Erin Lawlor's studio are
         published on her Instagram accounts, @erinlawlorstudio
         and @theerinlawlor.

p. 38   Discussion of Erin Lawlor's biography, both the
         developments in her work and their links to personal

events, was gathered from conversations with the artist, on Instagram, over email, in person and over Zoom.

p. 38 Two catalogue essays explore Lawlor's painting process, most specifically its physicality, the recording of the hand's movement and the specific processes explored in the studio. The first is Grant Vetter's essay, which appears in the catalogue to accompany the exhibition *Erin Lawlor* at Miles McEnery Gallery in New York, 3 February–12 March 2022. The second is Zoe Miller's essay 'The Fold', which appears in the same exhibition catalogue.

p. 39 Discussion of Erin Lawlor's stylistic developments, her process and specifically the role of edges in her work was gathered from conversations with the artist, on Instagram, over email, in person and over Zoom. The photographs referenced, of her studio and the edges of the canvas, are published on her Instagram accounts, @erinlawlorstudio and @theerinlawlor. Further reference photographs were shared directly.

p. 39 Discussion of Erin Lawlor's painting process and its connection to the operating theatre was gathered from conversations with the artist, on Instagram, over email, in person and over Zoom. The quotes *'leave everything there, all of yourself'* and *'I was here'* are taken from transcripts of these conversations.

p. 40 Ideas around Lawlor's paintings and their connection to the Baroque are explored in Grant Vetter's essay, which appears in the exhibition catalogue to accompany the exhibition *Erin Lawlor* at Miles McEnery Gallery in New York, 3 February–12 March 2022.

p. 40 Lawlor's discussion and quotation of Pier Kirkeby's painting and writing was gathered from conversations with the artist, on Instagram, over email, in person and over Zoom. The quote *'fundamental dishonesty of painting'* was taken from transcripts of these conversations.

p. 41   The discussion of the etymology of the word 'Baroque', and its connection to irregularly shaped pearls, was taken from various online sources, including the Wikipedia page on 'Baroque'.

p. 41   Lawlor's experience of lung cancer and its connection to her painting was something we explored in conversations on Instagram, over email, in person and over Zoom. I will remain forever indebted to the openness, vulnerability and generosity of Lawlor for allowing us to not only discuss such sensitive topics, but for being generous enough to read multiple drafts of my text as we tried to carefully think through the links between these experiences and her painting.

p. 41   The post-lobectomy photograph and quote *'Deep breath, ready to go under'* were published on Erin Lawlor's Instagram accounts, @erinlawlorstudio and @theerinlawlor.

p. 41   The discussion around how cancer cells reproduce is indebted to conversations with the writer and consultant oncologist Samir Guglani.

p. 42   The plastic bag found at the bottom of the Mariana Trench was something I first read about in a *National Geographic* article by Sarah Gibbens, 'Plastic proliferates at the bottom of world's deepest ocean trench', 13 May 2019.

p. 42   There are various scientific reports exploring the possible link between the ingestion of microplastics and the increased risk of cancer. A *Guardian* article, 'Microplastic found deep in lungs of living people for the first time' (6 April 2022), gathers together some of the research making the connection specifically to lung cancer.

pp. 42–5   Lawlor's quotes 'a *window of work*', '*doing heavy lifting . . .*', '*it felt so important . . .*', 'a *wild celebration . . .*', 'I was surprised . . .' and '*It really did feel like a conversation . . .*' were all taken from transcripts of our conversations on

Instagram, email and over Zoom. The wider discussions around these works were also informed by these dialogues.

p. 46   There are lots of journal articles and reports on foetal cells and DNA passing between the mother and the foetus. A *National Geographic* article by Ed Yong, 'Foetal cells hide out in Mum's body, but what do they do? (7 September 2015) usefully reports on some of the findings.

Chapter 4: Hatch

p. 53   The material on a blastocyst as 'a *hollow ball of cells*' and cells 'hatching' was cross-referenced across various online articles, but the specific quotes come from the online *MSD Manual*, in an article by Raul Artal-Mittelmark, 'Stages of development of the fetus'.

p. 56   It was during conversations on Instagram and via email that the artist Aimée Parrott told me about the work she was making while pregnant.

p. 61   '... *son of Jupiter and that Danaë ...*' and '*His rich golden shower*' comes from Ovid's *Metamorphoses*, Book 4, in the online English translation by A. S. Kline.

p. 62   '*saying that his colouring and his manner ...*' comes from Julia Conaway Bondanella and Peter Bondanella's translation of Giorgio Vasari's *Lives of the Artists* (Oxford University Press, 1991), p. 501.

p. 62   There are a number of brilliant books which address the rivalry between Venetian and Central Italian artists. Rona Goffen's *Titian's Women* is perhaps the most relevant in regard to the gendered nature of this divide. Johannes Wilde's book *Venetian Art: From Bellini to Titian* (Oxford University Press, 1981) gives a good account of the uniqueness of the Venetian approach.

p. 63   Discussion of Aimée Parrott's technique and processes owes a huge debt to the generosity of the artist in our dialogues on Instagram, email and over Zoom.

p. 63   Sarah Kate Wilson's review, in the *Journal of Contemporary Painting*, of Aimée Parrott's exhibition at the Pippy Houldsworth Gallery (August 2020) was instrumental in my thinking around traces and ghost prints in her work. The quotes '*sustained period of malleability* ...' and '*familial echoes bind* ...' both come from this review.

p. 65   Jack Smurthwaite's review 'At the western edge, with Atlas', published on Aimée Parrott's website, provides a good exploration of the role of serialisation in her work, and situates this within a wider discussion of its link to ecological issues of interconnectedness. His use of the word 'convergent' is developed in this essay.

Chapter 5: Eurydice

p. 75   Much of the thinking around Bracha Ettinger's work leant heavily on our conversations over email and Zoom.

p. 76   The photographs of Bracha Ettinger in her studio were published in Vol. 2 of the arts magazine *Nova Express*. It was a special edition focused entirely on Bracha's work. The publication also gives a comprehensive account of the role of the printer and archival imagery in her *Eurydice* paintings.

p. 77   Biographical details for the life of Cardinal Filippo Archinto were gathered from the Wikipedia article about him.

p. 79   The photographs of the Lodz Ghetto were published in Vol. 2 of *Nova Express*. A wider discussion of the role of these photographs in her work runs through the publication and was elaborated upon in my discussions with Bracha Ettinger.

p. 80 Brian Massumi's essay 'Painting: The voice of the grain', published in Vol. 2 of *Nova Express*, provides a comprehensive account of the role of the printer in Bracha Ettinger's *Eurydice* paintings. His quotes *'it takes time to stop time'* and *'frozen in the unoccupiable ...'* both come from this essay.

p. 80 Griselda Pollock's essay, published as an Introduction to Bracha Ettinger's book *The Matrixial Borderspace* (University of Minnesota Press, 2006), explores the role of touch in Bracha Ettinger's *Eurydice* paintings. Her description of Ettinger as a *'curator of wounds'* comes from this essay.

p. 81 *'pushes her back to death'* and *'irresolvable ambiguity'* are quotes from Judith Butler's essay, published as a Foreword to Bracha Ettinger's *The Matrixial Borderspace*. The essay also provided critical thinking around sight and death in Bracha Ettinger's *Eurydice* paintings.

p. 82 *'theory does not exhaust painting ...'* is from Bracha Ettinger's *The Matrixial Borderspace*, p. 93. The whole book provides a comprehensive account of her theory of the Matrixial Borderspace and in turn its relation to her *Eurydice* paintings.

p. 82 *'a partner in difference'*: ibid., p. 71.

p. 82 The idea of the womb as a borderspace, as a site of new psychoanalytical possibilities, is expanded upon by Bracha Ettinger in ibid., p. 71.

p. 82 The gaze, in relation to her *Eurydice* paintings, is expanded upon by Bracha Ettinger in ibid., p. 49.

p. 83 *'the artist's desire ...'*: ibid., p. 73. Here she also elaborates on desire as a Möbius strip.

p. 83 *'inflames the desire of my eye ...'*: ibid., p. 74.

Chapter 6: Under

p. 92 Simon Critchley's book *Notes on Suicide* (Fitzcarraldo Editions, 2015) is referenced in regard to his thinking, which pushes back on presumptions of suicide as an irrational act.

p. 93   '*thin ghosts*' is from Book 10 of Ovid's *Metamorphoses*, in the English translation by Mary M. Innes, p. 225.

p. 96   '*detached from its purely representational function*' is from 'Titian's blue', an article published in *The Lacanian Review Online* by Bogdan Wolf. The article was also useful in considerations around Titian's use of blue in his painting *Bacchus and Ariadne* (1523), particularly around blue and ideas of oblivion and the void.

p. 97   The observations on Jadé Fadojutimi's studio and the objects she surrounds herself with are based on the Tate Gallery short film *Jadé Fadojutimi's 5 Favourite Things*, which is available on the Tate official YouTube channel.

p. 99   '*I am always happy to shed ...*' is a quote by Jadé Fadojutimi which appears in the exhibition catalogue *Jadé Fadojutimi: Jesture*, co-published by Anomie Press and Pippy Houldsworth Gallery (2020), p. 47.

p. 100   '*Elasticity of imagination within ...*' and '*At times, my imagination has been taken ...*' are quotes by Jadé Fadojutimi which appear in ibid., p. 57. They are part of a longer piece of writing exploring her ideas around imagination.

p. 100   '*desperate to catch every breath*', '*now my paintings will just breathe*' and '*At one point I began inhaling ...*': ibid., p. 47.

p. 101   '*not hold us in place*' and '*living is truly remarkable*': ibid., p. 57.

p. 101   '*they become environments for me ...*' is taken from a Tate interview with Jadé Fadojutimi in 2020.

p. 101   '*I'm constantly walking along ...*': Jadé Fadojutimi, *Jadé Fadojutimi: Jesture*, p. 17.

p. 103   '*I want my gut to roll around ...*': ibid., p. 47.

p. 103   '*a gushing experience*': ibid., p. 27.

p. 103   '*I love to swell ...*': ibid., p. 37.

Chapter 7: Embrace

p. 112   The retelling of the life of Adonis takes Ovid's *Metamorphoses*, Book 10, as its source, particularly the English translation by Mary M. Innes, p. 225.

p. 112   Thomas Puttfarken's *Titian and Tragic Painting* was the most important text in guiding my thinking around the iconography and movements of the figures in Titian's *Venus and Adonis*.

p. 112   *Titian* by Charles Hope was particularly helpful in clarifying details and providing documentary evidence around the commissioning of Titian's *Venus and Adonis*.

p. 114   *'reaching out to all kinds of embryos'* and *'a theoretical condition'* are from an online article by Sadhbh O'Sullivan, 'What is super-fertility? It's not as straightforward as it sounds', published on Refinery29, 26 November 2021. The article is also more broadly discussed in terms of its description of hyperfertility.

p. 115   Dr Pragya Agarwal's research on unconscious bias; the best further reading on this thinking is her book *Sway: Unravelling Unconscious Bias* (Bloomsbury Sigma, 2020).

p. 123   The details surrounding the death of George Dyer were supported by details in Wieland Schmied's book *Francis Bacon: Commitment and Conflict* (Prestel, 2006) and by the Wikipedia article on *The Black Triptychs*.

p. 127   The idea of the body as meat and Bacon as a butcher is something Gilles Deleuze elaborates upon in his book *Francis Bacon: The Logic of Sensation*, translated by Daniel W. Smith (Bloomsbury Academic, 2017), p. 16.

p. 127   Martin Harrison and Rebecca's Daniel's book *Francis Bacon: Incunabula* (Thames & Hudson, 2008), has been a pivotal source in regard to research on the materials in Francis Bacon's studio. The book relies on the studio archives held by the Hugh Lane Gallery in Dublin, which has also been an invaluable source, particularly regarding the books Bacon had in his studio.

p. 128   '*photographs are very damaged by people walking …*' is a quote from Francis Bacon's interviews with David Sylvester, which are collected together in *Interviews with Francis Bacon* (Thames & Hudson, 2016), p. 45.

p. 128   '*renew them*': ibid., p. 14.

p. 129   The resemblance between the photograph of John Deakin and the ripped photographs of Michelangelo and the *Apollo Belvedere* is noted by Michael Harrison and Rebecca Daniels in their book *Francis Bacon: Incunabula*, pp. 30–31. The book has also been pivotal in terms of demonstrating the types of migrations that happen from source image to painting.

p. 130   '*a coagulation of non-representational marks*' is a quote from Francis Bacon's interviews with David Sylvester, in *Interviews with Francis Bacon*, p. 67.

p. 130   Bacon's connection to the late Rembrandt self-portrait is something Gilles Deleuze elaborates upon in his book *Francis Bacon: The Logic of Sensation*, p. 18.

p. 130   '*the body attempts to escape from itself …*': ibid., p. 17.

p. 131   '*a curtain where the Figure shades off into infinity*': ibid., p. 24.

p. 131   '*cosmic dissipation, in a closed but unlimited cosmos*': ibid., p. 22.

p. 131   '*O that this too too solid flesh would melt …*': *Hamlet*, Act 1, Scene 2.

p. 131   Michael Harrison and Rebecca Daniels cite various examples of where Bacon has used images from *Phenomena of Materialisation* as sources for his paintings. Notes on this appear in their book *Francis Bacon: Incunabula*, pp. 30–31.

p. 132   Notes on the controversies around Eva Carrière's experiments are indebted to a review of *Phenomena of Materialisation* on the website *The Public Domain Review*. The article is merely titled 'Phenomena of Materialisation' (1923).

p. 132   *'it was a marvellous photograph I have of grass ...'* is a quote from Francis Bacon's interviews with David Sylvester, which are collected together in *Interviews with Francis Bacon*, p. 183.

p. 132   *'practically fallen away'*: ibid., p. 183.

p. 133   *'dust seems to be eternal ...'*: ibid., p. 214.

p. 133   *'know about the lastingness of things'*: ibid., p. 214.

p. 134   *'nothing is behind the mirror ...'* is from Gilles Deleuze, *Francis Bacon: The Logic of Sensation*, p. 12.

p. 134   *'each day in the mirror I watch death at work'* is Bacon quoting Cocteau in his interviews with David Sylvester, ibid., p. 214.

p. 134   Martin Harrison's observation that a still from Cocteau's film *Le Sang d'un poète* (*The Blood of a Poet*) might have had a direct influence on Bacon's painting *Jet of Water* (1979) appears in his book *In Camera: Francis Bacon, Photography, Film and the Practice of Painting* (Thames & Hudson, 2005). The book more widely has had a significant impact on my thinking around the role of photography and film in Bacon's painting practice.

p. 135   *'that people have been dying around me like flies'* is a quote from Francis Bacon's interviews with David Sylvester, in *Interviews with Francis Bacon*, p. 201.

p. 136   *'Suppose the Figure had effectively disappeared ...'* is from Gilles Deleuze, *Francis Bacon: The Logic of Sensation*, p. 23.

p. 136   The notes on Baron von Schrenck-Notzing's investigation of Eva Carrière are based on a reproduction of the original publication of his text *Phenomena of Materialisation: A Contribution to the Investigation of Mediumistic Teleplastics*, translated by E. E. Fournier d'Albe (Kegan Paul, Trench, Trubner & Co. Ltd, 1923).

p. 136   *'undisturbed'* and *'her special faculty consists entirely ...'*: ibid.

p. 138   Notes on the police investigation into Eva Carrière are indebted to a review of *Phenomena of Materialisation* on the website *The Public Domain Review* titled 'Phenomena of Materialisation' (1923).

p. 140   '*I paint from remembered landscapes . . .*': Joni Mitchell in a letter to John Baur, published in *Nature in Abstraction: The Relation of Abstract Painting and Sculpture to Nature in Twentieth-Century American Art* (Whitney Museum of American Art, 1958) p. 75.

Chapter 8: Scatter

p. 143   Details around the Baader-Meinhof group and the subject matter of Gerhard Richter's *October* paintings were gathered from Gerhard Richter's website, which has extensive documentation of the work.

p. 143   '*The deaths of the terrorists . . .*' is a quote by Gerhard Richter taken from his website, in the wider documentation of his *October* paintings.

p. 143   The most comprehensive account and critical writing on the *October* series is in Robert Storr's book *Gerhard Richter, October 18, 1977* (Museum of Modern Art, 2002).

p. 145   The discussion of the Baader-Meinhof phenomenon is indebted to the Wikipedia page on 'Frequency illusion'.

p. 151   The photographs of Robert Rauschenberg by Jasper Johns were published in Ed Krčma's book *Rauschenberg/ Dante: Drawing a Modern Inferno*.

p. 151   The material on Robert Rauschenberg in this chapter is indebted to Ed Krčma's book *Rauschenberg/Dante: Drawing a Modern Inferno* (Yale University Press, 2017). It is also supported by the generosity and clarifications of Krčma in our exchanges over email.

p. 152   Details of Robert Rauschenberg's relationships with Jasper Johns, Susan Weil and Cy Twombly were sourced from ibid.

p. 152   A wider discussion of the links between Rauschenberg's compositional structures and the structuring of Dante's poem is explored in ibid., p. 20.

p. 153   *'depthless-deep'* is from Canto IV of John Ciardi's translation of Dante Alighieri's *Inferno* (Penguin, 2003), p. 53.

p. 153   *'Death-pale, the Poet spoke ...'*: ibid., p. 56.

p. 153   Ed Krčma gives a more extensive description of the landscape of Dante's seventh circle in his book *Rauschenberg/Dante: Drawing a Modern Inferno*, pp. 77–8.

p. 154   Krčma's *Rauschenberg/Dante: Drawing a Modern Inferno* provides the most comprehensive analysis of these works, including a detailed discussion of the transfer method and the manner in which Rauschenberg sourced his materials from mass media. The latter is a form of art history as archaeology, often involving painstaking research to link certain imagery back to its source and to then unpick possible iconographic meaning.

p. 154   Ibid., p. 20, discusses the link between Rauschenberg's continuation of a long lineage of adaptations.

p. 155   Ibid., p. 39, discusses the presence of Titian's *The Rape of Europa* in Rauschenberg's *Small Rebus*.

p. 156   The differing interpretations of Jonathan Katz and Ed Krčma regarding the figures and imagery beneath the red foot in Rauschenberg's *Canto XIV: Circle Seven, Round 3, The Violent Against God, Nature, and Art* can be found in ibid., p. 81, discussing the link between Rauschenberg's continuation of a long lineage of adaptations.

p. 157   The musical nature of the mark-making (and the nod to Cy Twombly) in Rauschenberg's Dante works is discussed in ibid., p. 17 and p. 53.

p. 157   *'the fact Rauschenberg selected images ...'*: ibid., p. 100.

p. 158   *'beauty is now underfoot ...'* is from John Cage, 'On Robert Rauschenberg, artist, and his work' originally published in *Metro*, Milan, May 1961.

p. 158   Ed Krčma goes into further depth around the hostile environment towards homosexual relationships in America in the 1950s, and the need for the Dante works to act as coded, safe spaces, in *Rauschenberg/Dante: Drawing a Modern Inferno*, pp. 81–3.

p. 159   Ed Krčma's analysis of Rauschenberg's work *Should Love Come First?* can be found in ibid., p. 74.

p. 159   Ed Krčma's analysis of Jasper Johns' work *Diver* can be found in ibid., p. 76.

p. 162   Details of the *sounds* coming from a black hole can be found on NASA's website in an article published on May 4 2022, 'New NASA black hole sonifications with a remix'.

Chapter 9: Skin

pp. 166–7   *'limits and materiality of the visible world . . .', 'the skin of the object . . .', 'the possibility to go beyond being'* and *'subtleties of Venetian light are at play'* are quotes from the texts accompanying the Anish Kapoor exhibition at both the Gallerie dell'Accademia di Venezia and the historic Palazzo Manfrin. They are also available in full on the Lisson Gallery website.

p. 169   The X-ray of Titian's *Venus with a Mirror* can be seen on the National Gallery of Art's (Washington) website.

p. 175   Maria Loh's book *Titian's Touch*, p. 224, gives a comprehensive account of the various fires across Venice in the 1560s and 1570s, the arrival of the plague in 1575 and the wider social and personal conditions in the final years of Titian's life.

p. 176   *Titian* by Filippo Pedrocco and *Titian* by Charles Hope both provide strong documentary evidence over the making of *The Flaying of Marsyas*. The latter, and Thomas Puttfarken's *Titian and Tragic Painting*, both provide illuminating discussion on the debate around Titian's late style and the level of finish in this and other paintings.

p. 176   *Titian* by Charles Hope provides a useful guide to the place that *The Flaying of Marsyas* and *The Death of Acteon* had in the *Poesie.*

p. 178   '*deep veins*': Ovid's *Metamorphoses*, Book 3, in the online English translation by A. S. Kline.

p. 178   Maria Loh's *Titian's Touch*, p. 232, references and discusses the validity of John Berger's musing on Titian stroking his dog while painting. Her entire book gives a wider deep dive into the role of touch in Titian's work.

p. 179   '*Why do you peel me out of myself?*': Ovid's *Metamorphoses*, Book 3, in the online English translation by A. S. Kline.

p. 181   '*for Weatherford, the story of neon . . .*' is from Francine Prose's exhibition essay, which was on display at the exhibition of Mary Weatherford's *Flaying of Marsyas* paintings at the Museo di Palazzo Grimani, Venice (2022).

p. 182   '*As he screams, the skin is flayed . . .*': Ovid's *Metamorphoses*, Book 3, in the online English translation by A. S. Kline.

p. 188   '*The mythical tortures of the lower everlasting time . . .*': Lucretius, *On the Nature of Things*, from the online English translation by Cyril Bailey.

Chapter 10: Crossings

p. 194   '*all human beings are mortal and natal*', '*infantile amnesia means that the rationale . . .*' and '*when we pay attention to infantile amnesia . . .*' are all from Alison Stone's article 'Thinking about one's birth is as uncanny as thinking about death', published on the website Big Think, 30 November 2019.

p. 197   '*an endless series of metamorphoses . . .*' is a quote by Cecilia Alemani from her interview with Marta Papini in *The Milk of Dreams* exhibition catalogue, 59th Venice Biennale (Silvana, 2022), p. 28.

p. 197   '*this means that the exhibition . . .*': ibid., p. 31.

pp. 198–9 The discussion of various artists' work from *The Milk of Dreams* exhibition was supported by exhibition texts, also collected together in the exhibition catalogue.

p. 200 *'We've heard it, we've all heard all about . . .'* is from Ursula Le Guin's essay *The Carrier Bag Theory of Fiction*, ibid., p. 418.

p. 200 *'since its purpose is neither resolution . . .'*: ibid., p. 420.

pp. 200–01 *'And hero, in Woolf's dictionary, is "bottle"'*, *'A book holds words. Words hold things.'*, *'how people relate to everything else . . .'* and *'arguments of some feminist critics . . .'*: ibid., p. 418.

p. 201 *'self-forming and self-sustaining are fantasies'*, *'a carrier bag for ongoingness'*, *'making-with'* and *'nothing makes itself'* are all from Donna J. Harraway's essay 'Sowing worlds: A seed bag for terraforming with earth others', in ibid., pp. 422–7.

p. 203 *'still there are seeds to be gathered . . .'*, Ursula Le Guin, *The Carrier Bag Theory of Fiction*, ibid., p. 421.

p. 204 Maria Loh's *Titian's Touch*, pp. 224–6, gives an account of the impact of the plague on Venice in the final years of Titian's life.

p. 204 A wider account of the impact of the plague on Venice during the final years of Titian's life is provided by the online article 'Renaissance lockdown: How Venice tried to control the plague' by Rosa Salzberg, published on the website History Workshop on 3 June 2020.

p. 204 The claim that Titian intended his *Pietà* for the altar of the Capella del Cristo was made by his early biographer Carlo Ridolfi in 1648. This is cited by Filippo Pedrocco in his book *Titian*, p. 308.

p. 204 Maria Loh's *Titian's Touch*, pp. 239–41, gives an account of the death of Titian's son and then Titian, including the transportation of his body.

Bibliography

Agarwal, Pragya, *Sway: Unravelling Unconscious Bias* (London: Bloomsbury Sigma, 2020) Alemani, Cecilia, et al., *Milk of Dreams* (Milan: Silvana, 2022)

Baur, John, *Nature in Abstraction: The Relation of Abstract Painting and Sculpture to Nature in Twentieth-Century American Art* (New York: Whitney Museum of American Art, 1958)

Brown, Patricia Fortini, *Art and Life in Renaissance Venice* (New Jersey: Prentice Hall, 1997)

Cole, Bruce, *Titian and Venetian Painting 1450–1590* (Boulder: Westview Press, 1999)

Critchley, Simon, *Notes on Suicide* (London: Fitzcarraldo Editions, 2015)

Deleuze, Gilles, translated by Daniel W. Smith, *Bacon: The Logic of Sensation* (London: Bloomsbury Academic, 2017)

Egmond, Florike, *Eye for Detail: Images of Plants and Animals in Art and Science, 1500–1630* (Chicago: Chicago University Press, 2016)

Ettinger, Bracha, et al., *The Matrixial Borderspace* (Minneapolis: University of Minnesota Press, 2006)

Falconer, Morgan, *Painting Beyond Pollock* (London: Phaidon, 2015)

Freedman, Luba, *Titian's Portraits Through Aretino's Lens*

(University Park: The Pennsylvania State University Press, 1953)

Goffen, Rona, *Piety and Patronage in Renaissance Venice* (New Haven and London: Yale University Press, 1986)

Goffen, Rona, *Titian's Women* (New Haven and London: Yale University Press, 1997)

Harrison, Martin, *In Camera: Francis Bacon, Photography, Film and the Practice of Painting* (New York and London: Thames & Hudson, 2005)

Harrison, Martin, and Daniels, Rebecca, *Francis Bacon: Incunabula* (New York and London: Thames & Hudson, 2008)

Higgie, Jennifer, et al., *Jadé Fadojutimi: Jesture* (London: Anomie Press and Pippy Houldsworth Gallery, 2021)

Hope, Charles, *Titian* (Hanover, PA: Chaucer Press, 1980)

Hope, Charles, and Jaffe, David, *Titian* (London: National Gallery, 2003)

Howard, Deborah, *The Architectural History of Venice* (New York: Holmes & Meier Publishers, Inc. 1981)

Humphrey, Peter, *The Altarpiece in Renaissance Venice* (New Haven and London: Yale University Press, 1993)

Huse, Norbert, Wolters, Wolfgang, and Jephcott, Edmund, translated by Edmund Jephcott, *The Art of Renaissance Venice* (Chicago: University of Chicago Press, 1993)

Hustvedt, Siri, *Mothers, Fathers and Others* (London: Sceptre, 2021)

Joannides, Paul, *Titian to 1518: The Assumption of Genius* (New Haven and London: Yale University Press, 2001)

Krčma, Ed, *Rauschenberg/Dante: Drawing a Modern Inferno* (New Haven and London: Yale University Press, 2017)

Loh, Maria, *Titian's Touch: Art, Magic and Philosophy* (London: Reaktion Books, 2019)

Lucretius, *The Nature of Things*, translated by A. E. Stallings
    (London: Penguin, 2007)

Meilman, Patricia, *Titian and the Altarpiece in Renaissance
    Venice* (New York: Cambridge University Press, 2000)

Miller, Zoe, *Erin Lawlor* (New York: Miles McEnery
    Gallery, 2019)

Millwood Hargrave, Kiran, *Orpheus and Eurydice* (London:
    Bloomsbury Academic, 2017)

Millwood Hargrave, Kiran, *Julia and the Shark* (London: Orion
    Books, 2021)

Ovid, *Metamorphoses*, translated by Mary M. Innes (London:
    Penguin, 1955)

Ovid, *Metamorphoses*, translated by Arthur Golding (London:
    Macmillan, 1965)

Panofsky, Erwin, *Problems in Titian, Mostly Iconographic* (New
    York: New York University Press, 1969)

Pedrocco, Filippo, *Titian* (New York: Rizzoli, 2000)

Pedrocco, Filippo, *The Art of Venice from its Origins to 1797*
    (Florence: Scala, 2002)

Penny, Nicholas, et al., *Metamorphosis: Poems Inspired by Titian*
    (London: National Gallery, 2012)

Puttfarken, Thomas, *Titian and Tragic Painting* (New Haven
    and London: Yale University Press, 2005)

Rosand, David, 'Titian and the eloquence of the brush',
    Artibus et Historiae, Vol. 2, No. 3 (1981)

Rosand, David, *Painting in Cinquecento Venice: Titian, Veronese,
    Tintoretto* (New Haven and London: Yale University
    Press, 1982)

Rosand, David, *Painting in Sixteenth-Century Venice: Titian,
    Veronese, Tintoretto*, revised edition (New Haven and
    London: Yale University Press, 1982)

Rosand, David, *The Franklin D. Murphy Lectures VIII: The*

Meaning of the Mark: Leonardo and Titian (St Lawrence, KS: Spencer Museum of Art, University of Kansas, 1988)

Roskill, Mark (ed.), *Dolce's Aretino and Venetian Art Theory of the Cinquecento* (Toronto: University of Toronto Press, 2000)

Schmied, Wieland, *Francis Bacon: Commitment and Conflict* (New York and London: Prestel, 2006)

Schrenck-Notzing, Baron von, *Phenomena of Materialisation: A Contribution to the Investigation of Mediumistic Teleplastics*, translated by E. E. Fournier d'Albe (London: Kegan Paul, Trench, Trubner & Co. Ltd, 1923)

Storr, Robert, *Gerhard Richter, October 18, 1977* (New York: Museum of Modern Art, 2002)

Sylvester, David, *Interviews with Francis Bacon* (New York and London: Thames & Hudson, 2016)

Tietze, Hans, *Titian: The Paintings and Drawings With Three Hundred Illustrations* (New York: Phaidon Publishers, 1950)

Vasari, Giorgio, *Lives of the Artists*, translated by Julia Conaway Bondanella and Peter Bondanella (Oxford: Oxford University Press, 1991)

Vetter, Grant, *Erin Lawlor* (New York: Miles McEnery Gallery, 2021)

Wilde, Johannes, *Venetian Art: From Bellini to Titian* (Oxford: Oxford University Press, 1981)

Wivel, Matthias, et al., *Titian: Love, Desire, Death* (London: National Gallery, 2020)

Wood, Paul, and Harrison, Charles, *Art in Theory 1648–1815: An Anthology of Changing Ideas* (London: Wiley-Blackwell, 2002)

Wood, Paul, and Harrison, Charles, *Art in Theory 1815–1900: An Anthology of Changing Ideas* (London: Wiley-Blackwell, 2002)

Wood, Paul and Harrison, Charles, *Art in Theory 1900–2000: An Anthology of Changing Ideas* (London: Wiley-Blackwell, 2002)

Wood, Paul, Harrison, Charles, and Wainwright, Leon, *The West in the World: An Anthology of Changing Ideas* (London: Wiley-Blackwell, 2002)

Wroe, Ann, *Orpheus: The Song of Life* (London: Jonathan Cape, 2011)

Acknowledgements

There are many artists and thinkers who have been incredibly generous with their time and expertise in the development of this book: Aimée Parrott, Andrea Bubenik, Ben Tuffnell, Bracha Ettinger, Ed Krčma, Erin Lawlor, Fiona Wollard, Matthias Wivel, Paul Joannides, Rebecca Daniels, Sam Guglani. Simon Palfrey and the studios of Mary Weatherford and Jadé Fadojutimi.

To my collaborators, who daily shift how I think about painting, poetry and the world. Most notably, for transformations, Simon, Mark, Andrea, Ali, Max, Pablo, Richard, Tally and Sam.

To my agent Harriet, who helped shape the book, including the gaps and spaces between things, and whose tender guidance is so deeply cherished. To David, and everyone else at David Higham. To Hellie, for support.

To my editor, Bella, whose deep intellect, vision and belief have been the engine behind the book evolving into its final form. To Lamorna, for patience, kindness and for making things happen. To Christine, and Linden for the Sisyphean task of copy-editing my work. To Francine, for the care of her proofreading. To Jamie for the wonderful cover design. To Sarah, for production wizardry. To George, Dan and the entire wonderful team at Granta, it still feels like a waking dream to be published by you all.

To Micky and the team at No 20 Arts, for their love and support of the artwork connected to this book. To Matt P., Paul S., Peter M., Stephen K. O. and Yasmina whose deep understanding makes my artwork possible. To Matt C. and Jeff, for rebuilding my studio after the fire.

To Alex, Amy, Andy, Chloe, Christiana, Dan, Ding, Elizabeth M., Elizabeth P., Freya, Harriet, James, Jessie, Jen, Jess O., Jess P., Kate, Katie, Kevin, Krystal, Lydia, Lucy, Mariah, Michael, Paul B., Paul F., Reece, Robin, Ros, Ruth, Simon S., Stephanie, Taz, Tim, Trees, Will and Zeba. For friendship, and being guiding lights in not only this book, but in our journey towards parenthood.

To Sarvat, my first reader, the person who helped us map a path through the darkness.

To Daisy and Matt, for everything really, but especially the offer of surrogacy, which still feels like the single most astonishing act of love.

To Zoe, Victoria, Ingrid, Zara, Charley, the team at the EPAU and the midwives at the JR, for making rainbows.

To Andrea, Martyn and my in-laws for your love and support.

To my mum, my sisters and wider family, for being my models for parenthood.

To the niblings, Tilly, Fred, Lilly, Emily, Leo, Pippa, Isla, Ted and Albie. For being the reason I knew I wanted to become a father.

To Luna and Marly.

For Kiran, for it all. For the words you helped me cut so the ideas could grow, for allowing me to write a book that shines light on what is and has been between us. For the babies we lost.

For Coral.